I0223245

ADVANCED PRAISE FOR

Leave Your Light On

It is with deepest appreciation that I share the following endorsements:

"*Leave Your Light On* is a truly inspirational tale of love and loss, extraordinary happiness, and profound sadness. Words and emotions leap off every page."

—**BOB IGER,** CEO The Walt Disney Company

"No matter when you encounter Shelley Buck, it is impossible not to be somehow transformed. Her raw willingness to trust, share and guide is all evidenced in this new memoir, where she recounts the unforgettable journey of love, struggle, loss and discovery, led by her son, Ryder."

—**THOMAS SCHUMACHER**
Producer of the Tony Award Winning Musical, The Lion King
President Walt Disney Theatrical Productions

"*Leave Your Light On* is one of the most honest, visceral, and inspiring books about love, loss, grief, and survival. There's no greater loss than that of a child, but Shelley Buck turns her loss into a gift for the world. She gives us the light of her son to carry with us as he inspires us to live our best lives."

—**JENNIFER LEE,** CCO Walt Disney Feature Animation

"*Leave Your Light On* is a beautiful and heartbreaking journey that highlights the lessons we learn from profound loss. Shelley and Ryder teach us that despite the weight of life's most tragic circumstance, wisdom, perspective and humor always find a way to rise to the top."

—**Kristen Bell**, Actress

"This searingly honest memoir in all its sadness, tragedy, and humor unleashes powerful emotional forces and a profound understanding of loss, and the cost of loving unconditionally. By turns poetic and pragmatic, but always illuminating, as Shelley shares her story we become part of the family on the journey from denial to acceptance, from pain to a deeper understanding of the true meaning of love."

—**Alfred Molina**, Actor

"A bittersweet and heart wrenching tale of a young man's journey into consciousness through physical hardship. It is a story that will inspire everyone to find the light in their own lives, and to cherish every day of the journey that leads them to it."

—**Peter Segal**, Director,
TOMMY BOY, 50 FIRST DATES, GET SMART

"Shelley's unfiltered realness made me laugh and cry in the same sentence, and reading Ryder's story makes me want to put down the sheet music and just JAM. Shelley's managed to show both the human and superhuman sides of herself AND Ryder. He is both a magical figure with an otherworldly poetic existence and an equally lovable and aggravating human being. I am changed forever by hearing Ryder's story, I feel like I know him."

—**Jonathan Groff**, Tony Award-nominated actor
for HAMILTON, FROZEN 1 & 2

"Take this journey with Shelley, Ryder and the courageous Buck family. You will come away forever changed. As I read the last page, I found myself infused with a kind of spiritual lightness and peace. It was as if Ryder, himself, had come and whispered in my ear, 'Life is beautiful. Live it large and let it sing.'"

—KRISTEN ANDERSON-LOPEZ, Oscar-winning songwriter,
FROZEN 1 & 2, COCO

"This amazing memoir comes straight from a mother's heart. Ryder Buck's light has hardly dimmed. In fact, it shines brighter than ever. You could warm your hands on it."

—CHRIS ERSKINE, Author/Columnist

"As a kid, I couldn't wait to grow up and be released from my parents' grip. As a parent, I cannot fathom letting go of my teenager. This book is undeniably relatable. It is a story about transition."

—JAMIE S. ROBERTS, Casting, Walt Disney Feature Animation

"… a mother's wrenchingly honest and beautiful love letter, not only to the son whose spirit sings to her from the other side, but also to the two sons and her soul mate who remain with her here."

—BRENDA CHAPMAN, Writer/Director

"Shelley pays beautiful tribute to her boy; in so many ways it's the story of Apollo, the god of music, truth and healing, as seen through his mother Leto's loving eyes."

—KEVIN LIMA, Writer/Director/Producer

"A profound and emotional book that is both life-affirming and uplifting, it details the inspiring journey of Ryder Buck, a creative, charismatic, and courageous young man, who lived life to its fullest and did so on his own terms in the face of overwhelming odds. Shelley Buck gives a brutally honest account of her sometimes contentious (but always nurturing and loving) relationship with her proud and independent son who refused to ever give up. Ryder's music and spirit live on in this extraordinary book, and the reader will come away better for the experience, feeling as if they'd gotten to know a unique and giving individual whose shining light left a profound impact on the world."

—**HOWARD GREEN**, Walt Disney Publicist/ Historian

"I'll never forget the moment I encountered the light that emanated from Ryder Buck. He was strumming a guitar on top of a popular hiking trail. He asked if he could play a song for us, and we experienced a lovely moment of live music performed by a stranger.

"This book is a beautiful tribute to a beautiful soul. It is a story of courage, hope, determination and tenacity, of finding light in the mountains and valleys of grief and reserves of strength within.

"Anyone reading this book will feel the warmth that defined Ryder, and will be touched by the grace that he and his mother discovered in themselves and each other… an unforgettable read!"

—**CATER LEE**, Broadcast Journalist

"'The light I'm about to share with you was earthbound, and now it's not'—Wow! Infectious and heartfelt, *Leave Your Light On* celebrates the extraordinary life of Ryder Buck and his passion for life, family and music. This unimaginable journey of a mother capturing her son's soul and spirit into a limited amount of words is remarkable. A true testament to the immense power of a mother's infinite love and devotion."

—**PETE DONALDSON**, Literary Manager

"To be close to the Buck family is to be forever warmed by their light. So, when the clouds block out the sun and the waves toss and the tide rips and you finally crawl your way to shore, come and sing a song of love, joy, peace, and hope with us around Ryder's fire...everyone is welcome."

—DR. WARREN BROWN

"A mother's celebration of a son she lost too soon and a deeply felt story of motherhood; a moving account of a son's search for health while trying to find who he was; and finally a quilt of memories of love between parents and children that lives beyond mortal lives."

—JOHN MUSKER, Director, Walt Disney Feature Animation,
THE LITTLE MERMAID, ALADDIN, HERCULES

"I loved reading this book. One sitting. It is unflinchingly blunt with honest reflection, cold candor, hot-blooded battles, and the never-remedied regrets that haunt to the grave. Shelley's simple profound words of wisdom are dropped so gently as if we all know these things to be true- motherly soft words full of hard truths.

"Through Ryder's generosity of spirit, he has shown how even the darkest streets can be lit with love. This book is about that illumination, his bright and warm loving light as if it was created expressly for us to spread love and joy alone. And most important for Ryder was making uplifting music. Ryder felt strongly, no matter what else you do with each day, be brave enough to be you. You have nothing to lose if you have won your true self and are following your own personal bliss. Life is short. But for him, you will find, just as long as it was meant to be, which was long enough to make a huge difference in many lives. Then and now."

—MIKE GABRIEL, Director, Walt Disney Feature Animation

LEAVE YOUR LIGHT ON

EAGLE'S
QUEST
PUBLISHING

Copyright © 2020 Shelley Buck

All rights reserved. No part of this publication may be reproduced, distributed, or transmitted in any form or by any means, including photocopying, recording, or other electronic or mechanical methods, without the prior written permission of the publisher, except in the case of brief quotations embodied in critical reviews and certain other noncommercial uses permitted by copyright law.

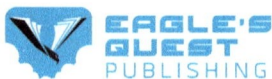

EAGLE'S QUEST PUBLISHING

ISBN
Paperback: 978-1-7344844-0-3
Ebook: 978-1-7344844-1-0
Hardcover: 978-1-7344844-2-7

LEAVE YOUR LIGHT ON

The Musical Mantra Left Behind by an Illuminating Spirit

Shelley Buck & Ryder Buck
with Kathy Curtis

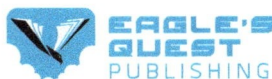

EAGLE'S
QUEST
PUBLISHING

I dedicate this book
to my first-born son, Ryder.
Thank you for having the courage
to shine your light,
no matter what.
It has given me the courage to do the same.

CONTENTS

FOREWORD

Chris Buck

Codirector, Disney's FROZEN and FROZEN II

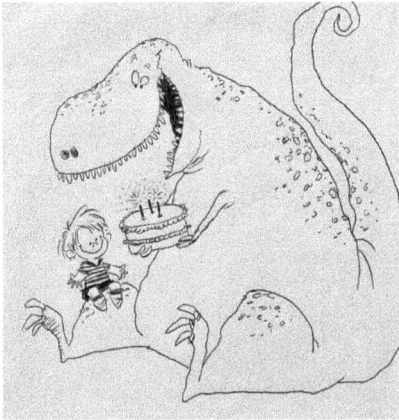

Ryder was a lot like me, with his quietly observant nature. I could almost hear the gears in his head turning from the time he was an infant as he took in the many experiences we excitedly shared with him. He seemed to love it all, as long as it wasn't too loud or didn't overstimulate him in some other way.

Each year, I would draw Ryder on his birthday invitation, capturing whatever it was he was into at that moment. For the longest time it was dinosaurs, but he loved all kinds of animals, so I never lacked for inspiration. Even his mischief and tantrums fed my muse.

Working in animation, I am drawn to stories that fill me with a sense of magic. Ryder's life story has been every bit as magical to me as the ones I've created for the big screen.

In the end, we think our first-born son told us a tale that is better than his mom or I could ever have created ourselves. Even though we gave him life, he gets all the credit for the magic and music he was determined to make.

Thank you for letting us share his story with you. We hope it inspires you to leave your light on.

PREFACE

The light I'm about to share with you was earthbound, and now it's not.

It came to life at Ryder's birth in 1990, shone brightly, flickered, and sometimes singed my lashes. It found its fuel in fits and starts, but it never dimmed. In the middle of the darkest passage, it became inextinguishable.

Ryder was an entertaining and exasperating character. As he grew older, his sense of mischief grew. Followed by wisdom. Followed by more mischief. His life was charmed, and yet it took unexpected turns that devastated us both.

Through it all, there was this light.

He understood what that meant long before I did. In fact, only in hindsight could I fully grasp what he was trying to show me his entire life.

How can we find our own light in a life that constantly distracts us from ourselves? Do only certain people have that ability? What role does our inner light—or that of our children—play in how we make our lives count?

These are the questions that drove me to tell this story. I could sum it up for you, but perhaps it would sound cliché.

If I let Ryder show you, instead, it might be like one candle's flame lighting another. It might leave you feeling the warmth of your own light in a way you never have.

He would love that. And I don't think he'd mind that I've shared both his charms and his flaws, so you can see how human he was while shining the light that made such a difference in this world.

We are so conditioned to see people from the outside, as though their behaviors and personalities are all there is. But when we can see the light within ourselves and others, it changes everything.

That is what Ryder knew—that living from a place of passion and purpose fills us with light both here and into the beyond.

If you're going through your own challenges, maybe Ryder can inspire you to see your situation in a new light. That's what he did for everyone who knew him. That's what he did for me.

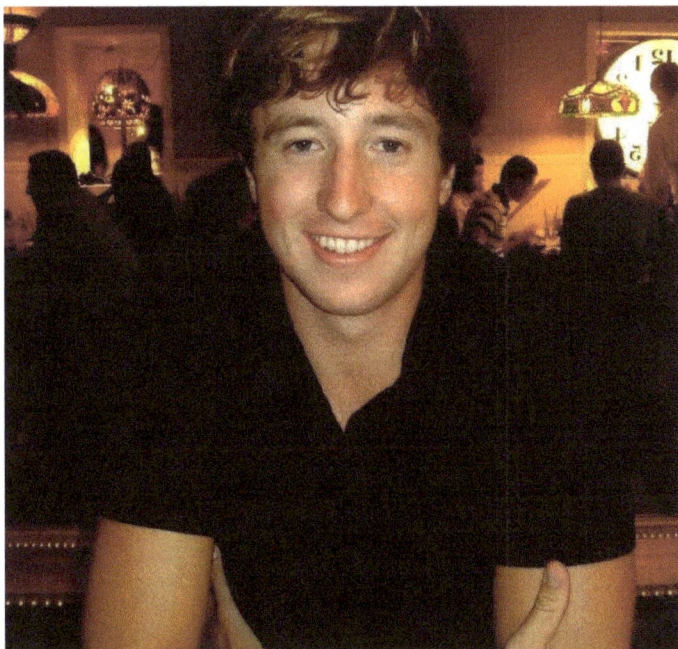

"See the light in others,
and treat them as if that is all you see."

—Dr. Wayne Dyer

MAGIC

My husband, Chris, and I met when we were in our twenties while working at Disney Animation. From the time we were young, we had both been captivated by the stories, characters, and visual delights that came from Walt Disney's imagination. We grew up wanting to make our dreams come true as Disney's animated films had inspired us to believe we could.

Chris' favorite was PINNOCHIO, the story of a boy growing up and becoming real. His love for animation started the day he sat in a movie theater with his parents and siblings to watch the film, and it never stopped. "When You Wish Upon A Star" is still his favorite Disney song of all time.

My favorite was SLEEPING BEAUTY. After seeing it, my mom made me a Sleeping Beauty dress which I wore all the time. I imagined myself having long blond hair, dancing through the colorful backgrounds, playing with the woodland creatures, and falling in love with my prince.

Right after college, I moved across the country to make my professional dreams come true, and I met my future husband and father of our three boys, Ryder, Woody, and Reed.

From the time our sons were born, we created magic in as many ways as we could. It was part of what drew us together, and we wanted them to enjoy it as much as we did. The leprechaun left green milk, green toilet water, and a touch of green food coloring on their toothbrushes. The tooth fairy tied a hair from my head (fairy thread) around a dollar bill and left footprints of glitter from the windowsill, across their foreheads, and onto their pillows. The Easter bunny unraveled a ball of yarn throughout the house and up and down trees in the yard, leading to baskets of goodies. Santa fills stockings to this day. Magic takes a lot of effort, but it's part of who we are.

A Valentine to My Three-Year-Old Ryder

Ryder,

My love for you is older than the dinosaurs, and more enduring.

It is fiercer than Tyrannosaurus Rex.

My love for you makes Ultrasaurus look like a tiny speck of sand.

It is bigger than the earth.

My love for you goes farther than the farthest star and back again, and around the world two times.

God alone knows the scope of my always forever love for you.

—Mommy

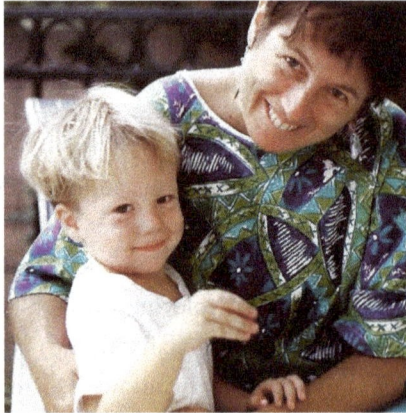

RYDER

FRESHMAN PSYCHOLOGY PAPER

"My Early Development"

I definitely feel I was blessed as a child, growing up in the loving and understanding environment that was my home. Though there were rough patches, for the most part, I don't think I could've asked for a better upbringing. My parents always exhibited an "authoritative" style of parenting, usually setting reasonable boundaries, but were not over-controlling. They were always very reassuring and if they had to say "no" to something it was always followed up by a valid reason (in their eyes, anyway). My mother and father are, to this day, very encouraging people, and they supported everything I did as a child, as long as it was a healthy activity.

I don't like the term "sheltered" because that's not an accurate description, but I was definitely censored from some things in the Buck household. For example, while a water gun might be allowed because of its harmless nature, Indiana Jones replica guns from Disneyland were definitely not, even if my slightly older cousin, RJ, was allowed to have them. I wasn't allowed to watch the MIGHTY MORPHIN' POWER RANGERS on television because of its "excessive violence." This never stopped me, however, from turning it on the minute I was left with our babysitter, Corina.

This would confuse my parents, though, when Halloween came around, and the only thing I wanted to be was the Blue Ranger. RUGRATS, worshipped by my peers and a staple of 90s culture, was also condemned by my parents for the snotty attitudes it portrayed. Despite all this "neglect" as a youngster, I managed to turn out as a fairly mild-mannered member of society, and apparently I was rarely a problem for my parents.

Siblings were a different story. Being a first-born had its advantages and disadvantages, and the sense of entitlement I had because of this showed absolutely no intentions of weakening the day I became an older brother. I was determined to bask in the glory of being my parents' favorite for as long as I possibly could, but this new creature that had forced its way into my world was ruining everything, and so began the competitive relationship I would have with my brother, Woody, for years to come. Life was a constant battle for attention, food, toys—you name it—and I had to come out on top, lest I'd be overshadowed by a younger, inferior being. That was my outlook on the situation for many years, and adding another brother, Reed, to the equation didn't help things much. However, the older I got, the more accepting I became of the coexistence I realized I'd have to endure.

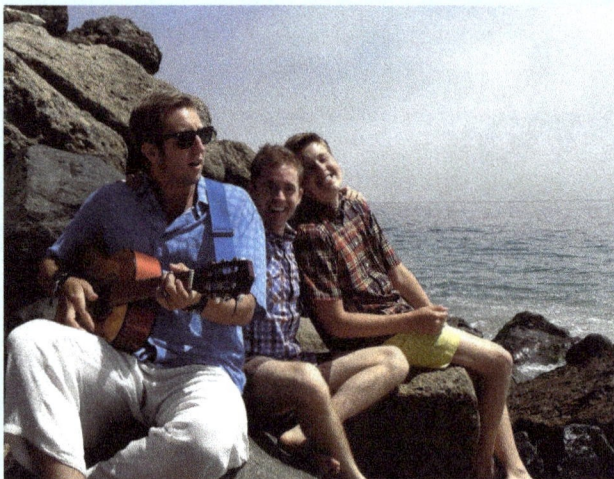

Thankfully, I have great relationships with both my brothers now, and going away to college strengthened those bonds, but for what felt like millennia, we were at each other's throats (not literally, I can count the number of physical altercations I've had with my siblings on one hand, but you catch my drift).

I honestly think that with a bit of luck, and if I stick to the methods my parents used with my brothers and me growing up, I can have an extremely successful family unit when I'm older.

RYDER'S EARLY LIGHT

I was an excitable bundle of ramped up energy anticipating Ryder's arrival. I felt like I'd entered a state of grace during my pregnancy and that my body was alive with a profound sense of wonder. Then he arrived in utter calmness, and I sat watching his eyelashes flutter for a full week before I finally took him out in his stroller for the first time. Even though we lived in a quiet neighborhood in Burbank with no through streets, I had an eerie sense we were enclosed in a bubble, walking in the middle of a freeway. I came home and thought to myself, "Traffic is moving so fast."

I've never forgotten the sense that I was transcending time that day. It was more than a sense, as time would reveal.

Ryder remained a calm baby who had to train me to tone down my excitability when it was too much for him. One night, as I railed against a news story on television, he started to whimper. When I dialed it back a notch, he quieted down.

As enthusiastic first-time parents, Chris and I introduced Ryder to big league baseball, theater, galleries, and zoos. Even as a babe-in-arms, he soaked it all up. This observant quality was a thread from his earliest days that carried into adulthood, helping him choose his friends and experiences from a place of careful discernment.

In preschool, watching from the side of the playground, he'd eventually focus on one child of interest to befriend. He chose well, as many of these early friendships lasted into adulthood.

When Ryder first started talking, he couldn't say consonant combinations. So he couldn't say *st*, *sp*, *tr*, and *mp*. One day, I picked up a dump truck and said, "What's this, Ryder?" And he said, *"Dumf*ck."* And I said, "Oooh, who's driving the dump truck, honey? Daddy?" He said, *"Daddy Dumf*ck!"* We roared. Well, I roared. I'm not sure Chris was thrilled, but Ryder's verbal antics would continue to keep us amused.

When Ryder was two years old, he pitched the only full-blown tantrum I ever witnessed when his brother, Woody, arrived. Throwing himself on the front lawn, kicking and pounding, he hollered, *"Take him baaaack!"* My calm little boy had a wider range of emotions than we knew. But he adjusted. And then adjusted again with the arrival of his second brother, Reed, a few years later.

When Ryder was five, we went on a tour of Disney Studios because one of Chris' colleagues was directing a dinosaur movie. He went over the storyboards with Ryder, who asked one question: *"Wait, why is the lemur friends with the dinosaur?"* He knew they didn't exist during the same time period. That wasn't the question. He was basically saying, *"OK justify this for me. I want to understand it. Where do their hearts lie?"*

By the time he entered first grade, Ryder already knew where his own heart belonged.

"Mallory's in my class, too!"

"You like Mallory?"

Big smile and twinkling eyes. *"Yessss."*

"Tomorrow is Wee Willie Winkie day and everyone's wearing their jammies to school."

And as Ryder was quick to point out to Chris, *"And Mallory's going to wear her nightgown!"*

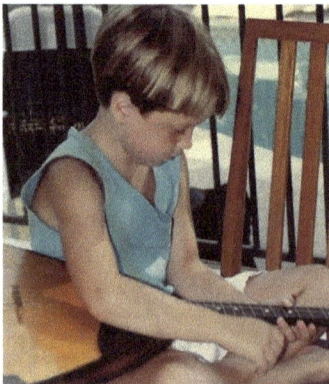

Ryder always enjoyed music. You could see that he was really listening, even as a child. When he was about six years old, I spotted him out on the patio. They were cutting down a tree next door, and he had a balalaika in his lap and a sad look on his face. I asked, "Honey what are you doing?" Ryder said, *"I'm playing a sad song for the tree."* He was all heart, that boy.

Ryder's tenderhearted kindness served him well with the girls from preschool on, and in turn, he was always sweet on someone. For homecoming his freshman year, he invited a girl to the dance. She had four girlfriends who didn't have dates, so he took them all.

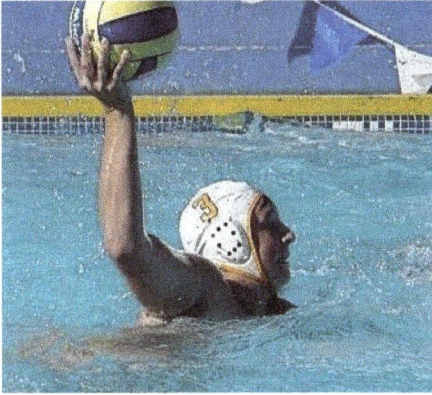

When he started high school, he moved into more physical activities—water polo, to be exact. A grueling, demanding sport, it focused his surging testosterone and taught him teamwork. Water polo got him out of his solitary endeavors and made a young man out of him.

Two things happened that led Ryder in an important new direction. First, he accidentally signed up for choir, which landed him in a very uncomfortable spotlight on stage. The other was playing Guitar Hero video games. He eventually got good at both, and by the time he was close to high school graduation, he got his first real guitar.

As he sprouted the soul of a troubadour, his ever-expanding emotional range was not always aligned with his spiritual growth. But we gave him a wide berth to grow the best parts of himself in a forgiving—or at least tolerant—environment.

Finding his passion for music led him to his best self. Soon he began to write love songs that flowed from his young man's heart. He would plop down on the end of our bed in the middle of the night and implore us to listen to his latest composition. Remarkably, he was egoless about this and urged us to give him honest feedback. We loved his humility.

There were other middle-of-the-night scenes that weren't so precious. Ryder started sowing a few wild oats with the newfound freedoms that came from having his driver's license. The loosening of restrictions on his curfew proved too much of a temptation, as we discovered one day around six in the morning.

I noticed light coming from under his door and popped my head in to say hello. His bed was undisturbed and the screen was out of the window! I called his phone, and to my surprise, he answered.

"I'm stuck at the beach. We're at the police station in Santa Monica."

He was with a girl I didn't know. The idea of a romantic walk on the beach in the middle of the night had apparently shut down their brains because they had left her car parked in the right traffic lane of the Pacific Coast Highway. The tow truck was just pulling away by the time they got back, which is when they were picked up by the police and taken to the station.

Confirming that both of them were safe and her parents were on their way, Chris and I got in the car for the long drive to the beach.

When he swaggered up to our car in his silky Playboy pajamas, I was so mad I couldn't speak. Something like this deserved a measured response. Should we take his car away? Obviously, but that didn't seem like enough. Then it dawned on me.

I had planned to take him to see the Rolling Stones. It was something we were both excited about, not just because they were my favorite band, but because we were going to share the experience as adults. So much for adulthood. I cancelled it.

We both cried over the loss, but I thought there'd be another chance when he was older. To this day, I deeply regret that decision.

Growing up in the world of animation, Ryder took his dad's work for granted until it finally hit home in a relatable way. The movies TARZAN and SURF'S UP brought skateboarding and surfing to life in his imagination. Ryder embraced each of them with enthusiasm, and after countless scrapes and bruises, he finally mastered both. He used the skateboard to get around campus, with his guitar strapped on his back, and made countless ventures to the beach with a borrowed surfboard.

Mostly, though, he and his guitar went everywhere together. He became obsessive about his music, just as he had been about his dinosaurs. He was still confused about what he should do with his life. When he asked my opinion, I told him to look in the mirror. It was strapped on his back.

Soon after, he found a music school and enrolled, finally feeding his soul with the instruction he craved. He fit right in and quickly gained a solid reputation with both teachers and fellow students. Ryder Buck was blossoming.

Beach jams beside a bonfire became his signature event. But he enjoyed performing anywhere, anytime, and he lived to spread the love that music brought out in him and everyone who listened. He formed a band made up of an ever-rotating cast of characters. As long as they met his "chill" standard and were willing to jam, they were in.

He was building an image. Flip flops, shades, sandy hair, and tan biceps. He saw his guitar as a "chick magnet."

RYDER

Sometime in high school, I picked up playing the guitar. I'd played violin when I was younger, and after failing miserably at that, I tried the piano. But my lack of interest, mixed with my seeming inability to find time to practice, led to my eventual exit from the music world altogether. This misfortune was remedied when, by some fluke of my own, I was placed in a choir class in seventh grade. I didn't sing…ever. My little brother, Woody, had always been the performer of the family, and I was perfectly content to let him hog the spotlight because I'd never shown any interest in it. That reminds me, being so wrapped up in writing about myself this whole time, I've neglected to mention the fact that I have two younger brothers. Woody, now a sophomore, loves the performing arts and musical theater, while Reed, now in sixth grade, shares my love of metal. I took him to his first concert, Iron Maiden, with some of my friends. But enough about them, this paper's about ME, right? So I was forced to sing for my school's seventh-grade choir, which I had absolutely NO intention of doing, but in a bizarre twist of events, I ended up completely falling in love with it.

Up to this point, the only artistic ability in my repertoire had been drawing, and it was my main way of expressing myself. But then a loving choir director and support from my family changed that completely. For the rest of my days at school, I always had a choir class, and I loved every minute of it. To this day, I am still a music fanatic and love nothing more than to sit down and mess around with my guitar.

So far, I'd say my life has been amazing. I can't truly complain about any one thing or say I regret much. Sure, everyone has had a missed opportunity they wish they'd taken and probably would if they could go back, but since we can't, why dwell on it?

Probably my favorite quote of all time came from a friend of mine who is wise beyond his years. I'd been having a hard week and stressing about a multitude of little things, and he just told me, "If you worry, you die. If you don't worry, you die. So why worry?" That quote has always stuck with me, and I try to live my life by it. Don't sweat the small stuff, make the most of every opportunity that presents itself, and you'll live a happier life...but that's just my opinion.

CANCER'S THUD

"I've got good news and bad news."

Life was humming along in the Buck household. Ryder was studying music at the Musicians Institute in Hollywood. Woody was studying musical theater in his sophomore year at the University of Michigan, fueling his dreams of performing on Broadway. Reed was a sophomore at La Canada High School, honing his own voice and acting chops in their excellent choir and theater programs. Chris was in his final year of production on FROZEN, his third and soon-to-be award-winning role directing animated films.

I had my fingers and heart in every detail of their lives as the hands-on wife and mother of this creatively driven family. I cherished my role of orchestrating our home life so they could be happy and successful. It fit me well. In between all the chaos, I was grateful for my jewelry design business into which I poured the extra love and creativity that I still had roaring through me after tending to their needs.

On this particular day, I was at Reed's high school painting graphics on a sports building. My phone rang in mid-brush stroke. It was Ryder, saying he had some good news and some bad news. Which did I want first?

"The bad news? OK, I have cancer."

"The good news? It's the kind that can be cured!"

"Wait! WHAT? Slow down. Where are you?!"

Ryder had developed a rash, which is what led him to see the doctor. During a routine exam, the doctor found some firmness in his testicle and did an immediate ultrasound. The ultrasound showed cancer, but as Ryder said, the prognosis looked good. He'd need surgery within a week to have the tumor removed, and then he'd find out about a treatment plan.

RYDER

So life's finally kicked me in the ass like I always knew it would. Bad news first: I have cancer. It's testicular, so there's a great chance I'll be fine and that's most likely the case (God willing). But say it's not His will. What then? What if I AM the unlucky 1 percent? What if the sand in my hourglass is finally running thin? Well, honestly, I wouldn't mind.

That's not to say I'm "giving up" or "welcoming death" or any of that morbid crap; I would hurt for my family and friends who would have to watch as one of their beloved brothers withered into dust, only to return to the sea from whence he came.

I'm very at peace with the idea of death. Sometimes it's slightly disconcerting to think about ceasing to exist in the world we know…but honestly, I would welcome my fate with open arms. The only thing that actually gets me down about it ever is the hurt in others' eyes—it makes me feel almost angry that something I had no control over can hurt the people I love THIS much.

But I guess that's life…learning to deal with the hand we're dealt and accepting the things we cannot change.

From the Beginning

Ryder's surgery to remove the cancerous tumor was successfully completed one week after his diagnosis. While we waited to get opinions from oncologists and select which cancer center we'd go through, Ryder squeezed every last drop out of his days and nights, mostly away from home.

Though Ryder gave me little insight into these forays, I surmised from a sandy towel and a wet dog that he'd been to the beach. Since his guitar was always with him, I knew he was making music somewhere—either publicly on the streets of Pasadena, privately on a mountaintop, or with fellow students from Musician's Institute. One thing never wavered, though. He was never home to say *"good night"* or up early enough for a *"good morning."*

I found out months later that Reed had been terrified Ryder would die on the operating table. He lived with that fear alone, inside of him, which broke my heart. And this left me with the ache I would feel so often in the months ahead about just how limitless the depth of a mother's love is when faced with the unknown.

Learning that my 22-year-old son had cancer was scary. Learning my son had cancer just as he was beginning to sprout his wings into adulthood tested my every maternal instinct. I was not going to let any bad decision-making get in the way of his full recovery, but as the doctors told me again and again, he was an adult and needed to be responsible for himself. This made our journey as much about mother-son dynamics as it was about getting him through treatment and back to health. The lessons in letting go and setting boundaries provided many growth opportunities. But we were a tough duo, and I knew we'd make it.

Early on, Ryder didn't want to bother with the details of his condition, but he was willing to go where he was told. I was at every doctor's appointment. I asked the nurses endless questions, surfing the internet afterwards to fill out my cryptic notes. I'm sure there were groups I could have joined, but I didn't. This was a partnership between Ryder, his caregivers, and me.

I tried to share all the information I was gathering, but Ryder just yawned. He rejected my attempts to bring him up to speed, breaking up the car rides by playing music or changing the subject. This was how he wanted it, and I went along. I knew we had a precarious balance, and I didn't want to rock the boat.

I couldn't imagine wanting to plod through all the information I was gathering at his age, either. But reading and learning gave me a sense of control, and it became my therapy.

What foods are most beneficial? Which are to be avoided? I discovered that what made sense to me about nutrition didn't necessarily get support from the medical staff. But I also learned how many toxins were part of our everyday lives from lawn care to pest control to household cleaners, and I made immediate changes on that front.

Ryder already knew how important his sense of serenity was to his healing, so I tried to catch up to him by learning to meditate. Did I succeed? Well...

There are so many unknowns about this disease, but research allowed me to take the wheel in an out-of-control situation and feel like I was proactive.

Still, at this point, Ryder wasn't really interested.

Thanks to many knowledgeable friends, we were given excellent recommendations for care. We soon had a treatment plan and a better understanding about what we were facing. But first we would wait. For tests. For tests to be approved by insurance. For test results. For tests of my patience!

Buddha Boy

From the start, Ryder wore his need for spiritual serenity on his sleeve. He seemed detached, more solitary than usual, meditative. When he couldn't find the peace he craved at home, he picked up his guitar and left, often without a word.

According to Woody, he still drove like a bully.

WOODY

Whenever we went anywhere together in Ryder's car, I wasn't allowed to touch the stereo. He drummed his fingers in time to the music on the steering wheel, never keeping a firm grip, which made me nervous. His use of the accelerator and brakes was jerky. It felt intentional, macho, and cocky. All of this pissed me off, and I didn't want to go anywhere with him, even though he was often my only form of transportation.

This charming dichotomy was only just beginning. Cancer does crazy things to a soul.

Like the night after surgery when Ryder blew up like a caged animal. He demanded the keys to the car, insisting he had to *"get away from this house, this town."* Us?

I put my foot down—no keys. He was livid. This put us both in fight mode. Then I switched to logic. He'd been through surgery not even 24 hours earlier. Wasn't some rest called for here? Then came the tears, and I finally heard him. He was desperate, and that got through to my heart. Against everything in my protective role as a mother, I could see we had to move forward in this battle—and it had to be on his terms.

I told him he couldn't run away from his condition, but I gave him the keys anyway. He stayed out all night. It hit me like a rock when he mentioned feeling impotent. I saw the car keys as his only form of control in an out-of-control situation and said a quiet prayer as he left.

It was exhausting. This whole exchange had taken place just as I was climbing into bed. I was sure I'd never fall asleep that night, but Chris talked me down. Maybe it really was the best thing for Ryder. How must he be feeling? He'd experienced a profound surgery for a young man. He needed to reclaim his manhood, his independence, his strength.

He must have been wondering *"why me?"* He must have been terrified. But I never heard him utter those words.

Ryder's apology, and mine, the next morning brought us closer to seeing that we were in this together. Hugs ensued. It wasn't going to be easy, but it was clear we had each other's backs.

RYDER

CANCER JOURNAL

I went off on Mom and Dad last night. I shouldn't have, but I basically yelled at them—trying to get them to understand why I wanted to get out. I would take back so many things if I could rewind time...but I have the most understanding parents I know. They got that I was feeling distant and slightly dehumanized by the cancer and the isolation it brings along with it.

Help is always something people should appreciate for the sheer kind-hearted gesture of it, but sometimes you JUST WANT TO DO IT FOR YOURSELF.

Not-So-Buddha Momma

Though I would have liked to escape this part of my life by drinking, I knew it wouldn't help.

In the old days, I'd have run from the anxiety I was feeling by reaching for a glass of wine. I knew, though, that there was nothing so bad that drinking wouldn't make worse. I just had to wait for treatment to begin, for Chris to be home so I had a partner in this, and for Ryder to come home where I knew he was safe. Waiting was excruciating. And this journey seemed to be all about waiting.

There was nothing to do, and yet I felt like I had my finger in the dike.

MICK

Longtime Family Friend

Holy crow Ryder…talk about getting a hot poker up yer arse, dude—you got it sideways! I'm truly sorry you're going through all this but Halle-flippin'-lujah they found it so early and acted so quickly. Is medical marijuana still legal? (Just KIDDING, Chris and Shel!) And you can thank your lucky stars treatment has come so far—back in the old school days when we went to class in caves and wrote using hieroglyphic math symbols with primitive chisels on the walls, back then when people even said the word "cancer," they'd whisper it like you'd had your car repossessed or like you'd been diagnosed with crazy. Ask your old bat mom…"Old Raptor ShelRae" remembers how it was. Those were the days. I can still remember your mom and dad around the campfire eating legs of wild boar, picking fleas out of each other's hair.

All right, Ryder, I'm going to close and will be thinking about how strong and amazing your support system is because you know Old Raptor ShelRae has already chewed off God's right ear with her instructions and demands. And ya know what? I believe God probably listened to her and is God-speeding you all the way back to the pain in the ass you were before all this came down. God bless and deliver you to health.

Medical Details

A friend asked that I post some of the details of Ryder's specific condition. I realized that "I have cancer" is like "I want ice cream." What flavor? How many scoops? Sprinkles?

Doctors told us it was choriocarcinoma. The numbers were high enough to positively identify cancer, but much lower than they might have been. There were also indicators for other possible types of cancer: small nodes in both lungs and suspicious lymph nodes in his pelvic area.

The pathology report showed Ryder's tumor was 95 percent embryonal, 4 percent choriocarcinoma, and 1 percent yolk sac. I really couldn't translate any of that, but for those who could, there it was. For the rest of us, beware of the internet. It can be scary.

Cancer's Coed Campus

Ryder decided on the oncologist who Chris and I also liked. I don't think it hurt that the grounds of his hospital felt like a college campus and was populated by young people (i.e., girls). He would eventually settle in with his guitar on the patio, making it feel as much like home as possible.

We felt we could breathe again, as this doctor came so highly recommended by several friends in the field. How lucky we were that we knew people who knew people!

Ryder's doctor said it was stage IV cancer, so there would be continuous lab work to monitor all his levels as they proceeded. They set him up for three cycles of chemo, and each cycle would include one week as an inpatient and two weeks as an outpatient. The plan would be to finish the week before Thanksgiving. We could smell the turkey dinner from there!

Food Becomes Our Medicine

Almost from the day we shared what was going on with our circle of family and friends, we began to receive the most delicious home-cooked meals delivered to our door. My friend, Sally, coordinated the whole thing and checked with us first to make sure there were no dietary restrictions. So even though I knew it was coming, I was overcome with tears the first time a friend showed up and handed us a meal across the threshold.

This went on every single day for the next nine months.

Reed thought he was getting takeout every time the doorbell rang, and new smells permeated the air with the promise of a delicious surprise. This kept my family fed AND happy. If home-cooked meals were a treat for their man-sized appetites, they were a relief for me because I didn't miss cooking.

It was one less thing to manage, and I already sensed my Wonder Woman cape was going to be threadbare very soon.

VIEW FROM THE PENTHOUSE

Ryder started chemo on Monday, September 17, 2012.

He had bounced back from his surgery and was feeling fit. On the surface, we were just following orders: packed, prepared, punctual.

As I drove, Ryder sat quietly in his own world. But under my calm exterior (I was taking my cues from Ryder) was a raging river of trepidation. How sick would he become? How quickly? I could only guess what he was feeling. I noticed he'd worn his championship water polo ring, which usually sat safely in his top drawer. It thrilled me that determination and grit were some of the tools he had packed for this foray into the unknown.

After we got him checked in and had his lab work done, we ate lunch on the patio while he played his guitar. His room on the ninth floor came with a view of the helipad and the setting sun behind the LA skyline. It was ironically idyllic.

He was scheduled as an inpatient for that week with the caveat that if he was climbing the walls and making the nurses crazy, he could ask for a pass to come home and make ME crazy. He saw that week as time off to read lyricists' books, write music, and play his guitar. And of course, keep his fans updated on Facebook:

> *So forward now is where I go*
> *Headed straight for the unknown*
> *Running towards the coming storm*
> *With only love to keep me warm.*
> *Catch you on the flipside!*
>
> *Peace & Love, Ryder*

Ryder's philosophy, which he shared with his nurse, was, *"The buffalo runs into the storm, spending less time in it."* I was impressed and hoped he would be able to maintain his perspective. Friends who had been through similar treatment told us what to expect, so I knew the buffalo might get lost.

I learned over time that some of the warnings we got from others who had been through their own cancer storms were too specific to their own experiences. Broad generalizations were more helpful to me, like remembering to back off and let him be in the driver's seat or making sure he got some exercise each day to help him sleep through the night.

A friend's son who had been through chemo made a personalized, artistic barf bucket for Ryder. It was a very sweet gesture of support, but Ryder wanted no part of it. It was too soon. He wasn't sick, yet. Much later in the process, however, that bucket would become attached to Ryder's arm.

On day one, we focused on settling in. Ryder curled up in bed and feigned sleep. He was passive, cooperative, and quietly curious. I was grateful. At least he wasn't fighting these first steps. We'd packed everything we could that would bring him comfort: His favorite pillow, his books, his guitar. If he'd have been younger, we'd have brought his blankie.

That evening, I left him to sleep, perchance to dream.

RYDER

Cancer Journal

Drip...drip...drip. The metronome-like click of the clock's hand lines up perfectly with the steady, plodding drip of the tinted liquid filling the bag at my bedside.

How did I get here? Memory recall brings back flashes of last-minute packing and the arduous commute through the sea of parked cars that is every LA freeway. This morning wasn't it? All those sweet smells and the comforts of home seem to melt away around me, preserved now in the far reaches of my mind, engraved in my soul. Only now are they being replaced all around me by the low hum of multicolored machines, the air cool and sterile, smelling faintly of pharmaceuticals. This is my home for the next week.

Vampire Hours

My midnight rambler was no different in the hospital. He typically started his days after Chris and I went home in the evening, sleeping well into the next day. I didn't mind because what mother doesn't love the peace of watching her child sleep?

On the very first night, a new doctor on duty thwarted his attempt to go outside and play his guitar at 12:30 a.m. Ryder could never keep anything from me for long, so he told me about it—almost proudly—the next morning. I think he got a kick out of it. I feigned mild disapproval but was secretly a little pleased that his spirit seemed undaunted. He was not a rule follower, and I admired that fire in him.

The next night, Ryder was seen doing Pilates at 11:30 p.m. in the lobby. The hospital staff frowned upon this. It didn't take nurses long to "get his number" and begin monitoring his activities. No matter how much his soul longed to play a concert to the stars out in the courtyard, if he was connected to his chemo drip, it was not happening.

Ryder's antics would butt heads more than once with his treatment. He honored the spirit of the law, just not the letter. But between my vigilance and that of his army of professionals, we kept things moving in the right direction while he nurtured his sense of well-being.

Why Was I so Tired?

With little to do while Ryder slept, I fretted and occupied myself with research, which led to information on cooking oils, filtered water, and vegetable juicers. Sitting idle in the middle of cancer wasn't an option, but I'm not sure if my friend, the internet, hurt or helped.

Even though I was not the one with poison coursing through my veins, this was exhausting. I kept asking myself, "Why?" All I did was sit all day, while others looked after his every need. I fetched coffees and smoothies, listened to him play his guitar, carried bananas and water bottles on his forays outside, and sat. Perhaps, I was so exhausted because I wasn't really breathing.

On our last night in the hospital, I packed up his library of books in anticipation of moving out. We bathed our dogs so there were no germs on them. The house was clean, and the fridge was stocked, so home looked like comfort from my perch in his room.

Home

Soccer.
No nurses.
The service sucks here.

~Ryder

As the doctors predicted, fatigue set in shortly after we got home. After pushing through a couple of late nights, a swim, and a hike, Ryder decided an afternoon nap sounded good. He woke up to terrifying nightmares and mouth sores, which doctors predicted.

Reed came home sick, and he and I both ended up on antibiotics. The thrill of the surgical mask wore off quickly for Reed, so we had to restrict him to his room. Wiping everything down with disinfectants also got old. What a circus.

It soon felt like Alice Through the Looking Glass. "Curiouser and curiouser."

Not Home

After those first couple of days at home, Ryder turned into Tigger, bouncing with energy and enthusiasm. He felt so good, he wanted to go camping. That was both the good and bad news of it. With low white cell counts, no cellphone reception, poison oak, and jagged rocks to climb, I was concerned.

This was payback, I thought, for when I was his age and skipped out the door to go skydiving. My mother said goodbye to me with tears in her eyes, certain she'd never see me alive again. Sorry, Mom.

I called Ryder's nurse about camping. She emailed his doctor who was in Berlin. His response was, "You will have to suppress your maternal instincts at times and let him be a man. It may be hard."

That was an understatement. He went, and I worried. I had to remind myself that nature is therapeutic. Solitude is where enlightenment happens. An invincible spirit is exactly what Ryder needed for this battle. I just wished he wouldn't have taken it to the streets—or the mountains—quite yet.

Letting Go

I tried to get Ryder to his outpatient treatment on time the last week before his second round began, but I failed. I hated being late, even though this was his cancer and his journey.

He got up late, even with my persistent prodding. He was dragging his heels, taking extra time with his shower, indulging in a languid breakfast, spending time with his dog. Tick. Tick. Tick. As the clock marked the minutes, I became more and more twisted, biting my tongue, breathing deeply, and reaching for patience.

After all, I kept my days open to care for him. My jewelry design business went on hiatus. I only saw friends when they dropped off meals or came to visit Ryder. My waking hours had been turned over to his ever-changing needs, and I was on call 24/7.

But I was constantly reminded that I had to let go and let him own his journey. This was part of the process, and I had to learn it.

So back to my computer I went—to my research, to my diversions. They kept me from dwelling on the fact that I was actually helpless.

Beanie Shopping

We went straight from the infusion room that day to the mall for hats. There was a pile of hair in his lap before they even unplugged him, which he donated to the birds outside. I felt sad for him, and those clumps of missing hair from his head made it more real for me. Then his attitude put me at ease. He was philosophical about his hair and vanity. He seemed to embrace the process entirely.

If this was how he was facing adversity, he would be fine through whatever else life threw his way. I imagined the strength and confidence that would come from this experience both in self-knowledge and through the conversations he would, no doubt, have with God.

That night he went to a Dodgers' game. His white cell counts were very low, and I'm sure Dodger Stadium should have been on his list of toxins to absolutely avoid. Just thinking about those bathrooms made me cringe.

Oh, well, maybe I'd dip him in chlorine the next morning.

Our Funny Bones

Humor was how we dealt with a lot of things in our home. Chris knew Ryder's sense of humor would help him in the coming months, and I could tell Ryder was starting to appreciate his dad's eye for the absurd.

"So that's how he stays so mellow—everything is funny to him," Ryder observed the morning after an evening visit with Chris.

That night, Ryder wanted to go outside to get some fresh air, then proceeded to run sprints on the grassy field until he almost passed out. Ryder started laughing at himself—so hard, he couldn't stop. Even though Chris was more concerned than amused, it became one of their favorite stories.

Ryder Buck

Ryder was constant amusement for Chris, and Ryder knew it. He cruised through the halls, attached to his beeping IV, which he affectionately named R2-D2. He broke all the hospital rules by going outside where his chemo wasn't allowed. Our son found the fun in being insurgent.

In Chris' mind, Ryder was the main character in a hospital sitcom. And he would beat all the odds in the end.

RYDER

CARINGBRIDGE

:) Hey all,

Yeah, I'm finally writing something here on CaringBridge.org. :P Sorry if it seems like I've been MIA. I've read and loved every one of your messages.

I just want to start off by saying a HUGE THANK YOU (caps lock, ahhh yeah...) to everyone who's taken the time to keep up with my recovery and for all of the love, support, prayers, and positive energy being sent my way; I can feel all of it. :)

My camping trip was spectacular and exactly what the doctor (should've) ordered, as I now feel rejuvenated and completely refreshed after getting back to nature and back in touch with the Spirit, which I'd been craving as of late. I knew being by myself would freak some people out (*cough* I'm sorry Mom...) but I knew just how necessary it was for my mental health.

Physically I've been feeling 100 percent for the past couple of weeks, with no signs of discomfort, minus a few annoying mouth sores. But enough about those; out of sight, out of mind. Even after all of the drugs they keep pumping into me, I continue to feel fitter than I've ever felt. I'd like to attribute that to all of the good vibes people continue to send our way in all forms. The dinners have been incredible and have taken a huge load off of my loving mother. For that I am eternally grateful. Anything to keep her stress levels as low as possible these days...well, aside from my solo excursions, I guess. Ha ha.

I just want to reassure everyone that as dire as my situation may seem at first glance because of the connotations that inevitably go hand in hand with the big, bad "C-words" (Cancer and Chemo), I am going to be completely fine—and by Christmas to boot! That's REALLY a blessing, considering how small of a blip nine weeks is in the span of one's life.

That being said, I really don't want anyone to worry about me, as I, myself, have completely left worry in the dust. Yes, I have been diagnosed with a chronic, and in some cases, terminal illness. But I'm not going to die from this. :) I have complete faith in the amazingly talented staff of medical professionals we have been blessed to be put in touch with and continue exploring any and all alternative methods of treatment. I have no doubt in my mind that strong mental and spiritual well-being are essential to anyone's survival. Western medicines and the sciences that make cures like chemotherapy available to us in this day and age are a miracle in their own right. But they are only an important half, the yin and yang. And what good comes from separations?

I love you all, and I would like to express my supreme gratitude, once again, for all of the incredibly heartwarming support that continues to pour in from all sides. It means so much, especially to my family, who is doing their very best to deal with this in their own ways. Thank you for everything: The meals, prayers, heaps of information I never thought I'd need to know, healthy alternatives, friendly suggestions, smiles, jokes, and good vibes...all of it. It shows me just how much people care, and that amount of love warms my heart like nothing else can. I wish you all the best as I head right back out into the world (hand sanitizers in tow) to continue living my life.

Love you Mom. I'll be back before dinner. ;)

Peace, love, and light to you all,

Ryder

Send Him Baaaack!

As we came up on week three of round one of treatment, the peaches and cream days were over.

It was a family ordeal, and I couldn't pretend otherwise, even for his sake. It was Ryder's journey, but it affected all of us.

As a 22-year-old, he wanted control. But he didn't want to do the work to keep up with it all.

He needed to read the doctor's notes. He needed to make himself aware of the side effects to watch for. He was responsible for knowing the specific things not to take and contacting his doctor when symptoms appeared as stated in the directions he refused to read.

Initially, Ryder didn't want to immerse himself in the details. He handed me the job of feeding him the information in snippets as he headed for the door to Hollywood, to the mountains, to concerts, and God knows where else. All I asked was to know that he was somewhere safe when I woke up in the middle of the night and saw his empty bed—which didn't always happen.

I was giving this kid everything in my power to get him well, and he was giving so little back. On the one hand, I couldn't blame him. He was facing something I never had at an age when he was supposed to be out doing exactly what he was doing. I was terrified and frustrated, and I felt guilty about asking anything of him. And that emotional cocktail was exhausting.

Taking him back to the hospital the following Monday for a week of inpatient treatment would be a relief. At least I'd know where he would be sleeping and that he'd have great care. I would be 40 minutes away if he wanted me there. But from his cues, what he needed was to be alone with this and learn to handle it on his own.

OK, who was I kidding?

I tried to feel out a moment when Ryder might be receptive to the information and instructions I was gathering. Timing was tricky. When he wasn't in the hospital, he seemed to want to forget that any of this was real. Since we had to face it, I wanted to see signs that he was accepting it and taking control. It was very uncomfortable to be the reminder. I hated the role. I yearned for us to be a team.

Once, I addressed my frustrations to him. Surprisingly, he was open and compassionate. But the door quickly closed and he retreated into his private world again. A world of forgetting. I couldn't blame him. The needles were a sharp reminder, the fatigue, the confinement, all the things he wanted to shake off. I was lucky to find a moment to slip in a quick, "Your appointment is Monday at eight." *"Grunt,"* he replied.

Secrets

He kept some secrets, mostly about where he was going and when he'd be back.

I didn't dare ask. I was on thin ice, always. Unless I was offering food. That was always welcome, and we had some lighthearted banter around the kitchen island. So Ryder and I did this uncomfortable dance, rarely connecting, but always together.

Was this Ryder finding his autonomy? His independence? His manhood?

I knew I'd have to move aside for all of these things as they were part of Ryder's toolbox. And I was letting go, consciously, with concerted effort by degrees. But it felt more like having an arm cut off than a gradual loosening of my grip—and Ryder was wielding the ax.

But the truth is like a tennis ball you try to bury under rocks at the bottom of the pool. It always finds its way to the surface.

Bloop!

How do you spell the sound of a tennis ball breaking the surface from the depths of a pool?

I knew Ryder wanted to get away. I even cheered him on when he found a wolf sanctuary an hour from home where he could enjoy the solitude of camping without being completely alone. Aunt Leslie joined him to see the wolves and spend some time with Ryder. After she helped him set up his tent, she headed back home.

When he pulled in late the next day and showed me the pictures on his phone, there was a shot of the Golden Gate Bridge after all the wolf images. Bloop!

He laughed, and I freaked out.

"San Francisco was just a little detour north of the wolf sanctuary."

Six hours north, to be exact.

"I was gonna tell you eventually, Mom."

I found it so much easier when we could lay the truth out on the table and let everyone deal with it. But I was trying—really trying—to see how this might have been part of his healing. He was shoring up his castle walls and establishing his stronghold. It was a necessary, though uncomfortable, separation.

At the risk of stating the obvious, it was not like me to stand by silently on the sidelines doing nothing. I knew my dad was laughing his celestial ass off. We all get ours when we have kids.

Timing Is Everything

From the moment our children are born, parenting becomes a process of separation. The trick is rejoicing at each step they take on their own—even as they are walking away.

This got very murky for me as my son became an adult just as his life was visited by a scary and unpredictable threat. I knew he wasn't ready to handle it on his own, but he didn't know that yet. Our relationship might have experienced growing pains in the best of conditions, but this was the worst.

I was committed to making sure he lived. He was committed to living in the moment. We both needed to win.

RYDER

Eighth Grade Essay

The water is warm. I am a bottle-nosed dolphin, leaping and diving somewhere in the South Pacific. A year passes, and now I am a Tyrannosaurus Rex in the Jurassic Period, hunting down herbivores and viciously tearing them limb from limb before I devour them. Three more years pass, and now I am a wolf running with my pack and silently stalking a gigantic moose. Now I am the great American bald eagle, soaring the skies, searching for a rabbit or squirrel to be the unlucky next victim of my awesome power. I look down on the world, and I am the master of all that I see. I am a young man, named after the eagle, and ruler of my world.

I only want one thing out of life. I want to live life to the fullest. Not in a bad way, like taking drugs or getting wasted, but in a good way, like going on adventures, going to college, getting married, and having kids (which I've heard can be an adventure in itself.)

I would like to finish eighth grade with good grades at the end of the year. I would also like to grow my hair out, not too long, but just long enough. When I grow up, I want to graduate from USC with a master's degree, get a career that I love (even better if it's high-paying), and get married and raise a family. That is who I am and who I want to be.

NO MORE SHENANIGANS

When Ryder started his second full week of inpatient treatment, we met with the doctor first. In a pleasant but firm tone, he grilled Ryder about his shenanigans over the past two weeks. His disapproval was clear; his sympathy for me, subtle.

Ryder was respectful and behaved like a gentleman with the doctor, adding a chuckle for punctuation. He always made me proud of the young man he was becoming. He knew how to compose himself in an unfamiliar world, which was not of his choosing.

The doctor took a moment after Ryder left the room to ask, "How are *you* doing?"

I told him I was relieved to drop him off for the week, then I suggested he put a lock on Ryder's door and maybe leg irons.

Breakfast before check-in was a fiasco. I was particular about the food he ate and what he ordered was real, nutritious, and tasty. Ryder hated it. He threw his fork down in disgust between bites.

He just wanted sausage—NOT BACON—in his breakfast burrito. That's how he ordered it, and this place, the hospital commissary, wasn't getting it right. And he hated that Reed called his new dog "Yogi" instead of "The Bear." Then he switched gears and wrote something poetic about dewdrops on the grass.

RYDER

CANCER JOURNAL

:/ Just to clarify a few things...

Maybe I'm just too used to my favorite brand of breakfast burritos or accustomed to flavorful foods, but that breakfast burrito yesterday was anything but tasty.

Real? Yes, there was definitely something that resembled a burrito one might eat for breakfast sitting in front of me. Nutritious? Last time I checked, tortillas containing mass amounts of melted cheese and loads of bacon weren't on the list of "the healthiest things you can put in your body." I had originally ordered sausage, but hakuna matata. I knew I needed the nutrition from what little egg was present. That brings me to the questionable use of the word "tasty." Apparently, my dear mother is not nearly as picky about her food as she claims because these eggs, I can guarantee you, were rubbery, cold, and bland; they were basically devoid of any real flavor. How she stomached them, let alone tried to convince me to finish mine, I do not know.

I knew there were vital nutrients inside the eggs, so I made a concerted effort to consume what I could. The equally ineffective "hot sauce" was not much of a cover-up for one of the saddest burritos I've ever tried eating. First and last time I try out the breakfast grill... :/ You win some, you lose some.

About the dog: I don't care enough to fight with my brother over the name of our newest family member. But I'm sure we're all familiar with the feeling of being excited about something that is newly yours and then having that feeling taken away by someone else's reinterpretation of it. Especially when it's coming from your headstrong, "my-way-or-the-highway" teenage brother telling you, "His name is Yogi." OK Reed, call him what you like. To each his own.

That is all.

This cancer continues to be a personal battle for me, but I'm fighting it off successfully with laughter, positive forward thinking, and a faith that something greater than my own self has got my back 100 percent.

I do not pity my situation, and I don't want pity from others. This is a life-changing experience for me, yes. But it has only improved my outlook on life, and I know, in time, I'll be back to complete "normality" again. Hell, I feel normal now, minus the IV in my arm. So please don't treat me any differently than you normally would if I were to pass you by on the street last year. I don't want people worrying about me because as I said before, worry no longer exists in my psyche. To worry about me is to look down at me with sympathy. And while smiles are nice, too much of that sympathy can be suffocating. I repeat, I am fine. So instead of worrying, have faith (like I do) that I will be back to perfect health in no time. It is that kind of positive energy I need on my side right now.

Were it not for this robot I'm attached to for most of the day, I'd be out swimming, long-boarding, and even running, which until recently, has never been my thing. But change is good, running especially. I just wish I had the ability and the energy to continue that change here in the hospital. But I guess this is time for me to "just chill" and take a break from being overly active out there. Thank you all for your continued support and faith in my situation. Catch you all on the flip side. :)

Smoother Sailing

After the burrito fiasco, Ryder's second inpatient week was uneventful. I hoped once I took myself out of the equation, communications between Ryder and the medical staff would open up—and more importantly, between Ryder and himself.

Chris arrived one night to find him warming up his voice beside the fountain out front and got a brief concert. I was jealous. I also heard he made plans to play guitar and go for walks each day, many of which were aborted for the sake of long afternoon naps.

I took the time away from the hospital to reflect on our experience so far and felt infinite gratitude for the quality of Ryder's medical care. Between his envelope-pushing and my need to know the answer to everything, the confidence I had in his medical team was an immeasurable relief. We felt like VIPs.

Even though the boys were growing up, my normal schedule as a stay-at-home mom was full. I was involved with their education, their athletic teams, and their social lives. I served on the public schools' foundation board, decorating for events and raising money for the schools in our district. As a water polo mom, I designed suits, jewelry, and graphics for the athletic buildings. As for their social lives, our house was always full of music, swimming, and teenaged testosterone. I loved all of it.

I also had a life of my own including my business, my friends, and a bit of travel. I tried to orchestrate it all with the goal of having fun, raising responsible sons, and keeping Chris' home life as simple as possible.

Now as I focused on Ryder's needs, I could barely keep up with Reed's demands for attention or my jewelry orders, which left little time for self-care. Friends prescribed hot baths, long walks, and gym time, which I tried my best to do. But I felt guilty when I was away from the hospital and I felt guilty when I was at the hospital. I was stretched thin between my two stations and nowhere was relaxing.

What began as a nightmare had become a grueling marathon, but we had support every step of the way. Our friends and family gave us their love, whether it was edible, audible, visible, or ethereal. I was a grateful mama, and my boy would soon be home.

Home Again, Home Again, Jiggety-Jog

I was stunned by Ryder's strength of body, mind, and heart as soon as he walked through the door. Even though I was the one who brought him home, I could see him more clearly in his own environment where he immediately filled the space with his *Ryder-ness*.

The first thing he did was greet Bear with a long, playful rubdown. He teased our other little dog, Bambi, by kicking a soccer ball around in the house. That drove Bambi and me both crazy. He checked out the contents of the fridge, even though he didn't have much of an appetite. He took over the TV, while simultaneously reaching out to all his friends on his phone. Basically, he fully reclaimed the space, and it felt divine.

I attributed his amazing resilience to his youth and, in no small part, to the prayers and good wishes of our powerful circle. Some of his numbers were not yet at the recommended levels, but the cancer markers were declining. We were heading in the right direction, but there still appeared to be a few sharks in the water.

Ryder seemed to be doing well, though. Translation: I immediately had no idea where he was much of the time. He'd come crashing home in a day or two, ready for the couch. Just like the first round, Saturday was for stretching his wings, and then he'd be horizontal all of Sunday and Monday.

Once home, he surfed the web, pulling up his favorite artists, TV shows, and friends' messages. I tried to imagine his days if we were still in the dinosaur ages of my youth. He'd have been climbing the walls. Yay, technology.

He spent a few days in his couch/bed/couch rhythm. I felt like I was watching from the bleachers, not really relaxed, ever vigilant, ever ready. And I was painfully aware he hadn't played any music all week.

The Bear stayed close.

Kryptonite

Apparently, they didn't give Ryder enough outpatient chemo to kill him in his third week. Or maybe it was the steroids that had him so energized.

He wondered aloud as he was bouncing off the walls, *"Why doesn't everyone do this all the time?"* Ummm...

Against the odds and all predictions, and even as he swung wildly from one extreme to another, he felt well. Whatever it was, he discovered he liked mornings, something he'd been missing for the last few years. It was new to have him with us before noon.

During this time, I could count on him to pound down a fresh juice cocktail every morning with berries, spinach, beets, ginger, and eye of newt. Then he was back to the guitar and going on political rants.

Ch-ch-ch-chaaaanges

The weight loss and hair loss were incidental and impermanent. The most remarkable changes were internal. Ryder was gaining newfound maturity, the kind some find in having their first apartment or world travel. For him, it was through discovering his own vulnerability.

I noticed his need for a serene environment as he moved further into his healing journey. He spent more time in his room or in the back yard with his dog, rarely sitting down to watch TV with the family. Just like young Ryder, who quietly played and observed from the sideline, I finally realized how challenging our energetic (read: chaotic) household had always been for him.

Ryder's deepening appreciation of life filled him with gratitude, optimism, and the joy of hard work. He visited Reed's water polo practice at 6:30 a.m. to share words of encouragement as the team headed into playoff season. He made plans to play guitar for cancer patients at a local hospital. Those things filled me with love.

His spiritual life exploded, too. He worked to define the concepts of the greater good, creative force, and God, which made for rich conversations. He decided the eternal question is, *"Why?"* And the answer, he found, was what you do with the hand you're dealt. I couldn't help but anticipate some enlightened lyrics.

As for me, I still put my internal life on hold so I could be hyper-observant. But I was undeniably changed by it all.

Are We There Yet?

According to projected timelines at our first meeting with the doctor, we were two-thirds of the way through treatment. Was that a light I saw? I was trying not to expect anything. I knew nothing was certain, but it was hard not to hope.

Ryder went hiking the morning before returning for this third inpatient week. I knew he was preparing himself mentally. I hoped it would be the last time he'd have to do so. We'd get the big test on Monday that measured the cancer markers. I couldn't wait because I loved numbers. They were such a simple, clear unit of measure.

RYDER

CANCER JOURNAL

*This really isn't as bad as everyone lets themselves make it. I feel it's so easy for us to let **possibilities** of what **could** happen to us (a.k.a. potential side effects) take over the way we think, and in doing so, let worry run our lives.*

*Really, though, we **create** our reality with the way we think about things. If we hear something unpleasant and think of it as an oncoming evil that we can't avoid, we doom ourselves before even facing the challenge ahead.*

*On the other hand, if we look at the positives of all things and only at what can be gained from a potentially horrific experience, we take the good from it and let the bad slip right off our backs. Yes, I have cancer. What can I do about it but take the steps necessary to overcome it? True, I **could** bemoan my situation and wallow in self-pity, as I let my ever-present fears run wild within my heart and make a mess of my mind. OR I could see through the "poor me" way of thinking that only leads to self-destruction and let the love from the Spirit take me over and do with me what I know it will. Faith brings with it an incredible sense of knowing, which is different than hope. When you **see** your reality in front of you and believe in **your own** inner truth, that truth will manifest itself before you.*

Trevor visited me today after he got a call about my situation. What an awesome friend. That guy has truly got my back, and a friendship like that should be treasured. The time he spent with me just "shooting the shit" and reminiscing about old trips and people we've known undeniably helped to lift my spirits and bring me inner peace.

*Others stopped by in the morning when I was fairly tired and useless, but their presence didn't do the same. Their faces held an unshakeable doubt, and that's something I don't need to dampen my reality with right now. **No time for doubt—only supreme faith.***

Sleep set back in sometime around Dad coming and going, and his presence is like that of a Buddha or God himself. My father is an incredible human being in so many ways, and I hope to the Almighty Spirit to someday be as centered and carry half the calming presence he takes with him everywhere.

I've been truly blessed by the love and support and people in my life that help flower my garden with each new day. I only hope I can somehow do the same for them and be a "shining light" to those around me (loving term my friend Allie used to describe me this morning). God, Jah, Spirit—whoever you are, please help me find the light I need each day and help me pass it on to those I come in contact with. Your light can never do harm.

Peace and love to all beings—kind, unkind, or indifferent.

EARLY RESULTS

As we waited for the lab results, Ryder's favorite nurses helped him get settled in for his final inpatient week. Things were quietly calm, giving me the chance to think ahead. Would I have the courage to get on a plane to go see Woody's college performance in Michigan?

Just as I began to doubt that I would, the results came in.

Ryder's white blood cells and platelets were back in the normal range with everything else moving in the right direction! The nurses patiently explained every little nuance of the numbers and gave me hope that this cycle would be his last. I wanted to dance!

That night I let myself cry for the first time since Ryder's surgery. Life's other channels kept blaring with Reed's roller-coaster world and Woody's circus. Things certainly didn't stop just because I was suspended in time, but I was breathing again.

I went to bed with the intention of falling deeply into sleep. The rest of it would have to wait.

More Sleep, Please

As the week wore on at home, Ryder slept more, too.

Meanwhile, Reed chipped away at what energy I had, challenging my stamina. Every day was a new debate. No matter how many ways I worked to accommodate him, he found a new bone to chew. Reed entered life at full charge; he was exuberant when he was young and miserable times 10 as a 15-year-old. I remembered this stage with Ryder and Woody, but Reed took it to a new level. Nothing I could do was right. Not food. Not driving. I knew nothing unless he wanted something. Then I was put to the task.

I was ready to throw in the towel and move to the hospital. At least the terrain there would be predictable, and the staff would always support me. Plus, I needed Ryder's music to soothe my soul.

Followed by Wake-Up Calls

Ryder called surprisingly early one morning from his hospital bed.

"I feel like I've been hit by a couple of buses, Mom."

I felt for him. My first instinct was to get in the car and head to the hospital, but we were trying to let him own this. Hearing my voice seemed to comfort him enough that we could be philosophical about what he was going through.

I told him it was kind of like a war after which the world just wouldn't look the same. He had faced his own mortality. No matter how hard or long the road would be after this, he'd always have a different kind of gratitude for the little things. Likewise, he'd have to be patient with those who treated small problems as if they were mountains. His new challenge would be to act with grace, along with giving back, being compassionate, and remaining centered. He got it.

As for me, I was taking a crash course in hands-off motherhood. Reed was ready to take the reins on his own life. He was close to having his driver's license, and I knew that would just be the beginning.

I kept thinking back to when they were learning to walk. The pediatrician reminded us to let them pick themselves up. They'd need that skill later, and there would be plenty of time to kiss the boo-boos afterwards. Letting them fall, though, was tough. It wasn't getting any easier, either.

Doing the Splits

With things looking up on the cancer front, there was no way I was going to miss Woody's play at college 2,200 miles away, so off I went with Chris and my mom to soak up all the magic our middle child brought to the world.

We gleefully cheered him on as he performed. Giving Woody every bit of my love and attention for four days was exactly what the doctor ordered. I needed the break and Woody needed us. But of course, I never forgot about Ryder.

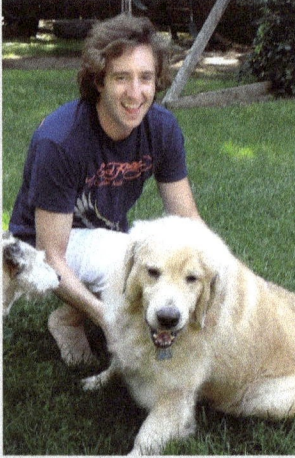

SUE

Longtime Family Friend

A big, goofy, Golden Retriever named "Bear" came into my life a few years ago. In my spare time, I have a nonprofit dog rescue. Once you realize that you can make a difference between life and death in a dog's life, you get hooked on saving them.

Driving to work one day, I saw a man walking a big, practically hairless dog. It was obviously miserable, walking slowly and hesitantly. I did a U-turn and said, "May I help you with your dog? I know a vet who can help him." The man replied, "Well, I wish you would!" Immediately I could tell that the man had lots of problems, and the health of the dog was not anything he could address.

A few days later, I took the dog to my vet. She is an expert at skin conditions and assured me he would be well in about four or five months. And sure enough, Bear slowly began to recover. But due to his age and skin problems, he could be considered unadoptable.

Not long after, I was sitting with the Buck family in their living room, listening to Ryder sing. Shelley asked me, "So what dogs do you have?" I rattled off my adoptable dogs, and then I said, "And I have a big Golden Retriever." Shelley and Ryder looked at each other and said, "We'll take him!"

Meanwhile, Back at Home

The barf bucket stayed as close as The Bear did while I was gone. The dreams left Ryder exhausted, even as he slept more than not. And his guitar sat idle.

The most noticeable change I saw after the weekend away was his bald, beautiful head. He had shaved the last few wisps, leaving him stylishly shorn. That's how I saw it, anyway.

Ryder talked to me about his dreams during his final outpatient chemo treatment. One of them involved a deadly snake in his hut on a tiny island. He separated the head from the body, but the head kept coming. He smashed the head and tossed it in the ocean, then he dove in and swam laps around the island. The symbolism seemed pretty clear and indicated strength to both of us. No matter what might lie ahead, we felt cautiously optimistic as the first step of this journey came to an end.

A Different Rhythm

We were two weeks away from follow-up tests to see how effective the last round of treatment had been. Life continued to ebb and flow in old and new ways. Ryder still had vampire hours, but he filled the daytime ones more thoughtfully. He met with his spiritual mentor, a long-time friend from our animation circle. He hiked. He ran out of steam and napped. He paid more attention to his diet. He wrote music and practiced for upcoming gigs.

Meanwhile, I gave thanks. It never left my mind that we were lucky to have found Ryder's illness when we did. His disease was aggressive, doubling every 60 days. But it also responded well to treatment when it was caught. And in Ryder's case, we did catch it.

I also thought about what it was and what it was not. Perhaps, some more tragic road had been averted by this detour. Maybe we had dodged a bigger bullet because we were nicked by this one. A greater mindfulness would certainly guide the choices we all made in the future.

With Thanksgiving just days away, I looked around at what normally would have been a winter wonderland of Christmas decorations. We (OK, I) go all out with a real tree in the living room, an aluminum one in the dining room window, a giant artificial one in the family room for the heavier ornaments, garland on the bannister and over the French doors, wreaths on the front and back doors, Disney figurines wearing Santa hats filling the shelves, a Santa collection crowding the bay window, and lights everywhere.

Chris always says it looks like Christmas threw up on our house.

And We Danced Around the Table!

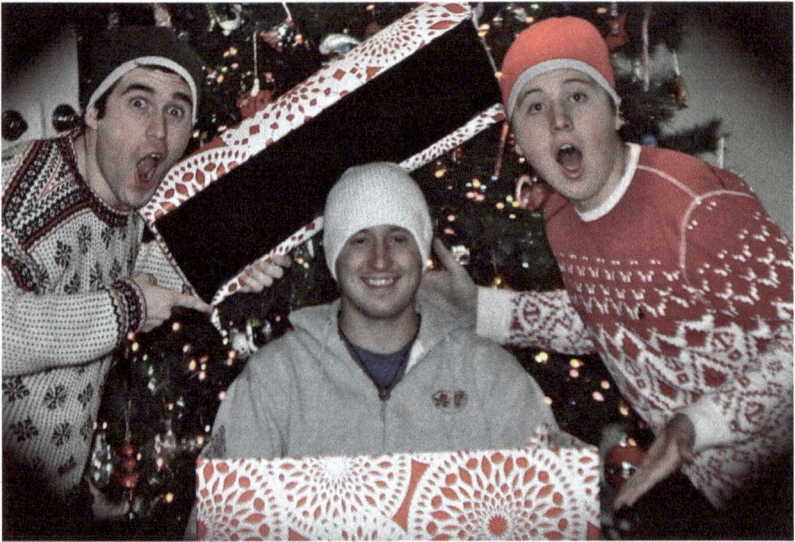

The entire family came together for Thanksgiving, which, more than ever, resembled a Norman Rockwell painting. The power of grateful hearts permeated the house. After all the ups and downs of the previous months, we were one relieved, happy family. Before the meal, we stood around the table holding hands, and one by one, we spoke our gratitude aloud. Then we danced…well, sort of!

Before the day was over, we took our Christmas card picture of the boys. They each sported beanies. It was warm that day in California, but everyone knew the beanies weren't to keep them warm (unless you counted brotherly love).

Later that weekend, Ryder learned his vitamin D levels were very low. He took off wearing shorts and flip flops to go snowboarding in the sun.

"I'll be fine, Mom."

I rolled my eyes.

"He hasn't always been this dumb," Chris said.

CHRIS

After the holidays, I went into my final year of work on FROZEN, and the last year of any film is the worst. Late hours take their toll on a normal life. But my life was far from normal with a son in the hospital undergoing chemo. Work was mentally exhausting, but the nightly hospital visits were emotionally exhausting. I was toast.

Ryder had just finished a round of chemo and was wiped out. At first, the side effects weren't as strong, so he bounced back quickly into his regular life—a life that had him away from home most of his waking hours. But this time was different. Ryder was around the house a lot more often.

I remember one special weekend afternoon. It was early December and the weather was beautiful. The pool had been heated to take off the chill, so I wasn't going to let this moment go to waste. I invited Ryder to join me, not really knowing if he was up to it.

I think he was in the water faster than I was.

We were both swimming laps, and even though Ryder's body was tired from the chemo, he was still a stronger swimmer than I was. We spent a lot of time in the water, talking about everything and nothing, as guys do. I mentioned the struggles at work, while he patiently listened. He talked about getting back to school, getting back to performing, and getting back to everything that would give him a normal life.

I got out and sat on a deck chair, while Ryder stayed in the pool, enjoying his second home—the water.

Then out of the blue, something, or someone, told me to soak up every second of this. This was a special moment—one that I may never have again.

I listened to that voice and was filled with gratitude for this time together. We continued talking, and I had a flashback of a young Ryder, splashing around the pool, doing exactly what he was doing now. As grown up as he was, he was still my little boy. And I was the luckiest dad in the world.

A HOLIDAY REPRIEVE

Everyone kept asking how Ryder was doing. That question had so many meanings, but here's what I knew.

His cancer markers were low. That was great.

His physical stamina was good. He was hiking, snowboarding, and jamming at the beach. He was sleeping more regular hours, which meant he was coming home before midnight. I didn't know if this reflected his energy level or maturity, but it was a relief either way.

There was so much meditation, study of the spiritual masters and philosophers, and introspection going on. The seeds had been planted for some serious growth, but I had a hard time reading this quiet germination period.

It was like he was starting over, finding his land legs. There was an uncertainty in him that seeped to the surface, a fragility of temperament, except when he was playing guitar. Then all was right with the world.

Still, if I was burdened by waiting for the final report, what must it have been like for him? I didn't know. We didn't make plans for the future. We all had faith that in the long term, all would be well. His hair would grow back, and his health and strength would return. But right now, we were stuck. Would there be more treatment? Could we travel over break when Woody was home? Should Ryder register for his final semester?

This was good training for being in the NOW, which is all we really ever have.

RYDER

The love feather, beaten and torn, sits straight up out of the sand to my right, remnants of a flight or a battle long since passed. The salt in the air tingles my nose, and I breathe in a deep lungful of all mother ocean has to offer. Her power is apparent in the ebb and flow of the swells of water dancing in rhythm before me. The pulsing beat syncs up with my heart, and I feel her pull, drawing me ever closer to that great divide—calling me home.

The sky is covered in a blanket of quilted clouds, grey and calm, warming my heart with a serenity rarely found elsewhere. This is where I'm most at peace, where man's rule ends and nature reclaims her hold on the world.

I can hear the distant squabbling of seagulls, completing the scene. Their calls are ones of desperation, a longing for something they still can't fathom. They long for an adventure out past the cliffs they call home, off into the divine sunset, wingtips stretched toward the glowing horizon.

Christmas Morning Came Early!

Two weeks before Christmas, we got the news that Ryder was CLEEAARRR!!!

I had to stop crying so I could drive us home from the hospital. All Ryder could say was, *"I told you so,"* over and over. He also said that he'd like to go to sleep and wake up with all his hair and realize this was all just a dream.

I was completely overcome with gratitude to God and for the grace we walked in even through the endless foggy nights of the last four months. I knew there was a greater purpose here that may never be revealed. Surely the music that poured forth from Ryder would reflect the underpinnings of this experience.

I was grateful for his life, for mine, for my other two sons, and Chris, who were all so precious to me. I was grateful for family and our dear friends, old and new, who had become our family through this.

I was grateful I never for a moment felt alone and that help I didn't know how to ask for just appeared. Or waited in the wings. Or was left in Tupperware on the doorstep.

Putting a Bow on It

Christmas brought Woody home from Michigan for two weeks, Reed was out of school, and Ryder's relatively quiet home front was invaded!

Woody was abuzz finding ways to reconnect with old high school friends; Reed and Ryder were both busy with friends, too. I was left trying to coordinate a meal or two where we could all sit down together.

When we did get together, there was so much music! Ryder strummed his guitar while Woody sang and Grandma Dot played piano. Even Bambi, the Chihuahua, kept time to the music, opening and closing her jaw to the rhythm of Ryder's guitar. We all got such a kick out of that, especially Chris, whose lap she always found when he could finally be home for some much-needed family time.

The presents we bought for one another that year were thoughtful, heartfelt, and generous of spirit. Our family traditions were even more fun and meaningful than usual.

Since my early childhood, we had spent Christmas Eve making enough homemade pizza to get us through the holiday. Friends and family gathered around the island in the kitchen to help. Each of us took a role in the production by making sauce, frying mountains of sausage, cutting and sautéing vegetables, and grating cheese by hand. Amazing smells filled the kitchen as the dogs hovered underfoot to catch any fallen bits.

On Christmas morning, we were still in our pajamas and eating leftover pizza as we read the Christmas story from the Bible, sang "Silent Night" with Grandma Dot on piano, and then dove into our stockings and gifts. The dogs were buried in paper and ribbons, and there was nothing organized about the mayhem that ensued, just a steady rhythm of "oohs" and "aahs." We even had stockings for the dogs, filled with rawhide bones and new chew toys.

But all the gifts took a backseat to the true gift of the season: Our health, specifically Ryder's. Christmas day had a special magic that year with a carefree, easy feeling we all shared. We were so immeasurably grateful, and we all breathed a collective sigh of relief.

We would have more tests and meet with the doctor again in March. For now, we were breathing the peace of God's amazing grace and opening our presents with gusto!

The Aftermath

As we got some distance between the shock of it all, we started to process the road we'd just been down with all its surprise twists and turns, potholes, and fallen trees. During it all, we just hunkered down and marched through the treatment. Now for the first time, we could look back and say, "What have we just been through?"

Ryder said he'd had enough coddling. I didn't think I'd been coddling him, but he was most certainly the focus of my attention for three and a half months. We put everything else on hold. We all entered that limbo with him and for him.

But like a wild animal released from his cage, he was soon gone.

Things seemed to go back to normal so fast. I tried to suppress my needs, but was a moment of shared joy too much to ask? It reminded me of Life of Pi when the tiger unceremoniously walked into the jungle when his story was over.

I longed to celebrate with Ryder, but his goal was to be free and move on, and I was inextricably tied to the cancer. I may have pouted on the inside, but outwardly I rallied and celebrated his freedom. My greatest joy was seeing him perform, and there was plenty of that to come.

GRANDMA DOT

A note to those who may be confounded by Ryder's behavior. His short temper and self-imposed isolation, his need for control over little things like which channel played on TV, what he ate, and how we treated his dog were all attempts to be at the helm of his own ship.

Ryder is experiencing, at a very young age, the complexities of the life-into-death phenomenon—usually reserved for those of us who feel ready to study the transition.

Routine family courtesies may seem trivial, even annoying, when they interrupt serious thoughts of a higher plane. When he comes to the other side of this experience, he will be a grown man, one of vision and compassion. I imagine him tending to cancer-ridden children with soothing vocals and playful guitar riffs accompanied by his dry, natural wit.

Right now, more than anything, he needs us to understand that his grumpiness and downright cussedness are simply outward manifestations of the frustration he's going through. He is being forced to meet the infinitely greater personal challenges that confront him in his young life—all ramifications of a known insidious killer, cancer. Scary, huh?

We know that this phase will eventually pass. He will overcome his sadness and disillusionment, reclaim his optimism, appreciate the heartache endured on his behalf, and make joyful noises around us once more. This much is true. We always need to be mindful of the bigger battle we are sharing with him and patiently "never mind" the small stuff!

Ryder's Celebration of Life Service

Presbyterian Church

Friday, November 1, 2013

3:30 p.m.

Reception at the church, followed by shared stories, videos, and music performed by Ryder's band

ONE DAY

RYDER, POSTHUMOUSLY

One day
Just like any other
Some day
this one or another
You will look and see that I am gone
(but did I really go?)
I beg of you, don't weep for me
Can't you see I'm finally free?
Isn't this what you would wish for me?
Please tell me now you understand
I'll reach out to hold your hand
All you have was all I had to give.
My time on earth was just as long
As it was s'posed to be.
I'll stay close to let you know
That I am always here.
My love, like yours, will never cease
Be gentle with yourself.
There's so much more to living
Just love your life and keep on giving.
I'll be here, I am not gone.
I'll help you all to carry on.

CHRIS

Shelley and I agreed we only knew about 25 percent of Ryder as an adult. We didn't really know what was going on out there. But as we've learned, he was inspiring others by the way he lived and connected with people. They sensed he understood what his life was really about.

ALLIE

A Close Friend from Musicians Institute

I find myself wondering all the time, "What would Ryder think about this thing, this person, this song, this crazy thought I had or thing I did?" I never had to pretend to be someone I wasn't around him. I could be fully myself: Spiritual and vain, kind and bitchy, generous and selfish, wise and incredibly ignorant. He gave me the freedom to be fully myself in his presence. He truly dug the duality of human nature, and he didn't try to hide his, either. We need more of that.

THE OTHER SHOE

In his follow-up exam with our internist in December, I requested full labs, just because. A tiny voice said it might be a good idea, especially since we weren't going to see the oncologist for three more months. The results that came in right after the first of the year raised concerns. Those concerns put Ryder on the fast track for more tests.

I thought this had all been too easy. Three months of hell and now more to come?

Ryder seemed content, so I took a lesson from him. Hakuna Matata. Que sera, sera. At least I had done all the fussing and renesting and detoxifying and supplementing I could imagine. We would have to see what Monday's test results showed.

He realized at that point that *"this will be a long road, with ups and downs."* That was the first time I had heard him accept his disease as a reality. His faith in his body's strength to heal, his doctor's care, and his God were strong. This was good. It kept us all from spinning out.

Meanwhile, he was moving forward with his music. He auditioned and was selected as a featured artist on the relaunch of MySpace Artists' Page. He recorded an interview for posting along with one of his songs. Monday came, along with the results that showed Ryder's cancer markers were up times seven to 35.2. This was not good, but it was far better than if we had waited until March to do follow-up tests.

The CT scan showed a 1.5 cm growth on one of his lymph nodes. They ordered a biopsy, and we waited for the insurance company to clear the request.

They would consider several of the following options after the biopsy:

1. A different cocktail of chemo.

2. Stem cell therapy. As I understood it, his clean blood would be held in a baggie while they super-soaked him with lethal doses of chemo and then quickly replaced his healthy blood.

3. Surgery figured in there somewhere, possibly after frying the thing in #2.

If there had been a choice, I'd have voted to rip the Band-Aid off quickly and go for the surgery. But it was not my Band-Aid.

Apart from the cancer, Ryder's pulmonary artery was enlarged, so they ordered an EKG. The doctor and nurse looked poised to catch me if I fainted, so I was guessing at the degree of their concern.

SHAINA

Woody's Actress, Musician Friend

Dear Shelley,

I know that I have often written to you in support of you and your family since Ryder passed, but I have never written to you about what Ryder means to me.

Ryder has impacted me in ways that even I can't fully understand. It is true that I only knew him over Facebook, but I began to feel such a connection to him through all the things that he would post. His spirit simply RADIATED, and I felt like I began to really know him just by seeing the positive way that he approached the world.

I remember distinctly the time I posted, "Never give up. Never surrender!" This quote from GALAXY QUEST sparked a fun, banter-y FB conversation between us which truly made me smile. He was a kindred spirit.

Shelley, I can't explain it, but I still feel so connected to him, even more and more as I read posts from his close friends and people whose lives he touched. I know that you won't think it's weird when I say that I feel him around me so often. I think about him every day.

I talk to him a lot actually. Anytime I am appreciating the beauty of the small moments of life or living the large epic moments, I always look up towards him and somehow know that it is the type of moment he would drink in and appreciate.

Ryder's Days

Filled end to end with music, Ryder spent his days jamming with new collaborators, laying down tracks for his first EP, and playing his guitar on the streets of Pasadena. This practice time with an open guitar case sometimes brought in gas money and was a great way to meet other musicians. One of them, Andrew, even earned a spot in his band and eventually a place in our home and hearts.

I was impressed by Ryder's initiative and drive.

With no one giving him an external structure for his days, he was organized, focused, and productive. There may have been an urgency to proceed before the next pause for treatment, but I didn't feel any desperation. After his biopsy, he even scheduled a jam session with new musicians in the afternoon. I was confident he would be fine.

Four More Rounds

Although Ryder's biopsy was clear, his cancer markers had tripled again in two weeks. He would have to have another brain scan, even though the earlier one had been clear. Something was making these markers go up fast, but they didn't know what.

He was prescribed four more rounds of chemo with a different cocktail this time. Over the next 12 weeks, he would alternate between inpatient care for a week and outpatient care for two weeks, four times. This would take us into the second week of April.

This treatment was more aggressive, so he would feel sicker. He'd lose his hair again. The tests would tell how well it worked.

Surgery was still a possibility. Doctors talked about a bone marrow transplant, but they said that probably wasn't going to happen. Still, I took note. In the whirlwind of it all, I completely forgot to ask about the EKG. Really, my tiny brain was on overload.

CHRIS

Often, when Ryder got home from the hospital, he'd just grab his guitar and head right back out again.

He was trying to make every minute count. It was as if he was shot out of a cannon after the chemo. We rarely saw him. I called him my vampire because it seemed like he slept maybe two hours a day and then he was off running. Maybe he recharged in his yoga classes or at the beach. Lord knows how he caught up on his sleep.

When he was out of the house with friends, he was such a warm and inviting person. But we didn't see that side of him much. Home was where he could let off steam. It was where he could kick a ball or yell, and it was fine because home was a safe place. And who knows, maybe we frustrated him some with all our hovering.

Outside our home, I'd hoped he was doing some nice things. Every now and then I heard about them. But I had no idea how deeply he was touching people.

HALEY

Ryder's Friend from a College Trip Abroad

Ryder brought me out of the darkness. He came into my life when I was searching for answers, full of anger and hate, and praying to be released from this life. But all that changed when I met him, and slowly but surely his philosophies, his attitude, and his love seeped into my life and began to transform me. It would be an understatement to say I wouldn't be who I am today had I not met Ryder. I am more grateful, kind, and considerate. I feel love more deeply, I see other people more clearly and compassionately, and I thank God for every day I get to live this beautiful life.

Wrapping Our Brains Around It

Ryder and I were both approaching this next phase differently than the last. He wanted to dive into a better cancer-fighting nutritional regimen, so we watched Forks Over Knives. We planned the food I would bring to the hospital each day. I doubted the hospital commissary would whip up an organic, gluten-, dairy-, and sugar-free menu.

"I want to know everything about what's going on in my body," Ryder said. *"I want to know, so I can understand it and write about it."*

That was a step. Acceptance. Curiosity. Being proactive.

As for me, I knew I had to take some of my undirected energy and put it into my own health and exercise program. From that point forward, I took my books and my gym bag wherever I went.

MAX

High School Friend

Ryder and I were home from college on Christmas break, and he had come over five nights in a row to sit in the hot tub. The next night he messaged me over and over, but I ignored it. I just wanted to have a night to myself.

Around 10:00 p.m., I walked into the family room and heard a noise outside. Ryder had come in through my side gate, turned on my hot tub, and was sitting in it, grinning. I walked out and said, "What the hell are you doing, Ryder?"

He said, *"Don't worry dude, just chill. Come here."*

He jumped out and grabbed some chocolate chip cookies, peanut butter, and jelly from his backpack. Then he hopped back in and started making chocolate-cookie-peanut-butter sandwiches in my hot tub! I couldn't help but laugh. So I grabbed my suit, got in with him, and ended up having a great night.

That's the kind of guy Ryder was. He would force happiness and joy on you. He wanted everybody to be happy and relaxed all the time, no matter what. I have to thank him for that and for introducing me to the PB&J cookie sandwich that I still make to this day.

Ryder Gets Curious

Ryder liked the hardwood floor of his corner suite in the hospital. There were three chairs, a couch, a coffee table, and a nice view. The doctor liked Ryder's location better this time because it was in the same building as his office. It would be easier for him to pop in. I liked that, too.

For the first time, Ryder asked about his disease. The doctor told him the cancer cells making his markers go up were likely free-floating, possibly in the lymph nodes and lungs. The doctor said he could wait until something was visible, but why wait? He was lucky to have a jump on it and would have better, quicker results if he moved now.

The doctor expected these four rounds of chemo to take care of it without stem cell replacement therapy. He then advised Ryder against skiing, camping, and surfing since emergency rooms didn't like to see low white cell counts while setting bones. However, he did expect Ryder to be up for his next music gig in two weeks.

To my surprise, I felt much more serene this time like I might melt into my chair as opposed to hover over it.

It didn't hurt that Ryder had decided to treat me to a rare, private concert. He was perched on the edge of his bed, one foot tapping the floor as he strummed his guitar and sang. Hospital robe, gym shorts, and IV tubes notwithstanding, he looked beautiful. And it was touching to watch the nurses pause in the doorway to listen before hurrying to tend to another patient. Just as I got completely lost in the sweet sound of his voice, the dietician popped in. We had been waiting for this.

It was almost comical (almost) to watch her face fall by increments. Gluten free, check. Dairy free, check. Sugar free, uh huh. Vegetarian? Hold on, kiddo.

As Ryder painted her into an ever-shrinking corner, she tried to entice him with options. Filet mignon and scallop kabobs? No? She left scratching her head.

Fifteen minutes later, the Big Guns came in. At 6' 6" Dr. Quinn towered over Ryder's bed with a looming presence.

"I have bad news," Dr. Quinn said. "I think it's great that you want to be a vegetarian, but now is not the time to start. After chemo is over and all four rounds are completed in April, then you can start. Right now, you need lots of protein for blood cell production and muscle strength."

I had never seen Dr. Quinn so firm, even through all the camping, surfing, road trips, and various other escapades. This time he was resolute: eat protein.

Ryder wasn't happy about this. He sulked.

I was relieved that someone with greater authority than I had was speaking decisively on the matter. Vegetarianism requires its own massive research, and I was not about to make a guinea pig out of him while we muddled through it.

Ryder's mood darkened as the day wore on. He was polite, but anyone reading energy fields would have seen a thunder cloud rolling in. I figured it had to be about more than just the meat thing.

I browsed through the handouts on his drugs, and aha! One of the side effects was mood swings. I was grateful to discover that information and excitedly told Ryder about it.

He was relieved to know what created the cloud, which made it easier to shake off. He promptly took a couple laps around the floor and played a few songs on his guitar.

"I feel better now, Mom," he said.

Music may be his best medicine, but it was also helpful for him to know why the mood swings were coming. Sometimes we just need to understand why things happen the way they do.

I stayed with him for that entire day.

As I prepared to leave that night, he promised not to do anything *"stupid."*

MOLLY

A Best Friend from High School

Ryder and I LOVED McDonald's shamrock shakes. We anticipated shamrock shake season months in advance, and we even counted down the days. When it finally arrived, we were both giddy as we pulled up to the drive-through window.

Ryder: *"Yeah, hey, we want two extra-large shamrock shakes... and let's get some fries too."*

McDonald's lady: "We don't have shamrock shakes this year."

Ryder slowly turned his head towards me. His face scrunched up and with fire in his eyes, he floored the accelerator and sped out of the drive through, screaming at the top of his lungs. I laughed so hard I cried!

Let Me OUT!

On his final inpatient day, Ryder started his chemo treatment at 5:00 a.m. If all had run smoothly, we would have finished up around 6:00 p.m. Unfortunately, there was a snag at the pharmacy, and no amount of barking from the Chihuahua-nurse could speed it along. I offered to summon my inner dragon as backup, but she managed to wrestle it from them with some of the chocolate hearts I brought in to thank the nurses for their long week.

We made it home just before midnight. At 11:55 p.m., Ryder was tucked in. But that night, he made hourly trips from his bed to the bathroom.

Whatever they had given him to stave off nausea worked while he was in the hospital, but it seemed to have worn off when we got home.

Back to the Hospital

He hadn't yet been home 24 hours, but the promise of relief pried him away from his pillow and me from my couch. It was a big step for him to ask to go back to the hospital.

On the ride there, we were mostly quiet. Ryder felt nauseous and didn't want to talk, and I sensed there was little to say that would make him feel better. Sometimes Pollyanna wasn't welcome. We just had to get there.

They checked him in so the doctor could observe him for 24 hours.

No matter what the hour, the nurses had their wands waving.

Me: "Are you cold, Ryder?"

Whoosh! A blanket appeared, and nurses tucked it in around him.

TREVOR

Best Friend Since Kindergarten

One of our favorite games to play as kids was one we dubbed "Rock Dodger." It started when we were nine or 10 years old during a family trip to watch the Chicago Cubs at spring training in Arizona.

The hotel where we stayed had a huge pool with an eight-foot deep end. Around the perimeter of the pool were rocks varying in size from pebbles to baseballs. We would grab a handful and throw them as high as we could above the deep end of the pool then dive under the water with our goggles on, looking up. If we had been close enough to the surface, we would have gotten seriously injured. But being several feet below the surface, we could maneuver our bodies around them like ninjas. The game was exhilarating and gave us an adrenaline rush. We played it whenever we went swimming and there was something lethal and dense to throw in the air over the water.

When we were 16, I had the bright idea to try it out in the shallow end of Ryder's pool. We threw the rocks up in the air, dove under three feet of water to the bottom, and looked at each other in a state of panic. We knew we weren't deep enough to even attempt to dodge them. The rocks came screaming down through the water and struck us all over our bodies.

We both surfaced and simultaneously said to each other *"f*** that!"* We never played "Rock Dodger" again.

Good News and Bad News

After being treated for nausea at the hospital, we were soon back home.

The bad news was that Ryder wasn't complaining; he didn't have the energy for it.

The good news was, we now had an entire pharmacy on our kitchen island. By evening, he was noticeably more comfortable. Though this round of treatment had been worse than the previous one, he did yoga and ate a hearty breakfast the following morning.

Still, there was a sense of shell shock in the house. Ryder was on edge, and his condition at any given moment was unpredictable. He stomped through the house, grunted his responses to my questions, and had little patience for Reed's antics. We were all ready to dive for the foxhole.

Only Bear was a constant, soothing presence.

Ryder and I started working on boundaries.

He needed to learn how to express when he'd had enough input, care, and company. And I had to learn how to leave the door open, becoming more of a low tide gently lapping at the shore instead of a crashing wave. This had been our dynamic since the crib. I was still working on it.

For the next couple of months, Ryder was up and down, and in and out. I didn't know how he would feel from one moment to the next. When he felt good, he spread his wings, but there was no predicting his stamina. He said something about being *"fragile,"* which is not a word I would have expected from him. It wasn't that he was saying, *"poor me,"* it was more like he was acknowledging his weakened body, mind, and spirit. He no longer seemed to think he was invincible, and that is something we all need to learn.

By January, the flu season was in full swing, and it was making me crazy. Malls and coffee houses seemed to be places teeming with bacteria.

But Ryder had been hooked up for eight days, and he was restless. Ryder had always filled his days and nights with the things that kept him happy and inspired. Even if he was tired, he wasn't built to be idle.

I just couldn't deny him the fresh air. Honestly, I couldn't really deny him anything. He had to find his own limits. I just didn't want there to be any hiccups in his treatment, like the bug going around flattening my strong, otherwise healthy friends.

Valentine's Day?

After a day of visiting with friends, Ryder finally got to have dinner with his dad. This was a rare treat since Chris was working long hours now that the movie was in the home stretch. Since it was Valentine's Day, they both made a special effort to be home at a reasonable hour.

Magically, the dinner our support team sent was one of Chris' favorites: Salmon with asparagus and a hearty salad. It was exactly what I WOULD have cooked if I were up to cooking.

Chris and I were used to his work keeping us apart during final movie productions, but I was really struggling this time around. The stakes were higher than ever, the family demands were more intense, and I was worried that something important was going to be overlooked. It was all too heavy to carry alone.

I got short with Chris, just like Ryder got short with me. We were all stretched to a place beyond reason, and reason often got lost. Chris is as steady a person as I'd ever met, and I needed that—but so did the most important project of his professional career.

There wasn't much romance on Valentine's Day, but somewhere beneath the guilt and resentment and fatigue and fear, there was love. Even if we didn't say it.

Hitting His Stride Again

Within a week, Ryder was busy cramming in his social life and taking long walks with his dog. I knew he was storing up good times for next week's long road. If the last round was any indication, it would take at least a week for him to feel good again.

His hair was starting to fall out again. It was small stuff in the big picture, but it was still hard. The challenge was to keep perspective. We did our best to keep our eye on the prize.

In five days, I'd travel to Ann Arbor for a couple of days to see Woody's college play. Then I'd be home for Reed's high school performance.

The following Monday through Friday I'd be at the cancer center with Ryder for his first of the next four rounds of chemo.

One day at a time. Was there really any other way?

MAX

High School Friend

Late one night, we were driving to Ryder's house when he suddenly yelled, *"STOP the car!"* I slammed the brakes, and he immediately jumped out and hunkered down by the side of the road.

"What the hell are you doing?"

"There's a baby raccoon. I think I can get him."

"Dammit, Ryder. What are you going to do when you get him?"

"I'll throw him in the back seat."

"Of my car? No way, dude."

"It's chill bro. Don't worry."

Ryder wanted that raccoon so badly, and all I could see was the raccoon clawing at us and passing on his very UN-chill rabies. I finally talked Ryder back into the car, raccoon-less. He wasn't happy. He only said two more sentences to me that night. *"Take me home,"* and *"I could have had him."*

The next day, I went to his house, bitter about the night before. HE was mad at ME because I didn't let him throw a baby raccoon in my car? I was determined HE would apologize to ME.

He came up to me with a big smile, gave me a hug, and said, *"One love, man."*

"Dammit, Ryder." I wanted a proper apology, but he made it clear that there was no reason to stay mad over a raccoon.

Ryder was always carefree. I continued muttering "dammit, Ryder" for years, but it was impossible to say it without smiling. You couldn't truly be mad at him.

I keep asking myself what to do now that he's gone. I think the answer is to live in the moment. Do what feels good, right at this moment, and share that love with others. I'm not suggesting picking up roadside raccoons whenever you please. I just think following Ryder's lead would do us all some good.

Ryder

FACEBOOK

You really want to know how I'm doing, Facebook? Well, after six stabbings and two failed attempts at setting an IV, round two of four is finally underway. Boredom seems to have its way with you in this place.

On a lighter note, words of wisdom I stumbled upon this morning:

> *"Humankind has not woven the web of life. We are but one thread within it. What we do to the web, we do to ourselves. All things are bound together."*

> *--Chief Seattle*
> *Duwamish-Suquamish Tribe, 1785-1866*

Choose to have a good day. :)

LUISA

Shelley's Friend and Partner in Her Jewelry Business

When Ryder began working at my little café, he was still a teenager, which is one of the most confusing times in life. As far as I could tell, his only challenges were related to that most elusive cappuccino foam, a bossy boss, and the unexpected attention from a crew of older girls.

I fondly remember one afternoon a few years later when Ryder came back for a visit. He had since faced challenges way more dramatic than cappuccino foam, and he offered the gourmand excuse of craving a fennel salad for his return. He actually seemed more interested in having a conversation, which is why our time together became a much-treasured memory.

The topic: How much we humans open ourselves to—or deny—the search for a higher power. It was pretty intense, and our perspectives were often not in total agreement. He, the way younger one by decades, was much more at peace, as if he had it all figured out. I, the much older one, was still rebellious and ready to raise any argument like a toreador's cape, red and inflammatory! We discussed how various cultures address, manipulate, and exploit that very concept and ultimately how personal and yet sharable all of that can be!

Did we finally come to a common agreement? Was that really the point? Possibly.

In the end, what I will always treasure is the TIME, the TIME that a young man gave me. Because for an older person, nothing compares to the TIME that a younger one is willing to share.

Thank you Ryder for your love. I hope to have matched it.

Luisa (a.k.a. the bossy boss)

Hump Day and Beyond

On Wednesday, during his second week of inpatient treatment, Ryder slept a lot, saying it helped pass the time. He admitted he was irritable, claustrophobic, and tired of his hospital room, even with its wall of windows. He snapped at me, then apologized.

We looked forward to a walk when he was unplugged later that afternoon, but when the time came, he wasn't up to it. On Thursday, he was pretty wiped out, too, but Friday brought renewed energy in anticipation of going home.

This treatment was a different animal than last fall. It was much more intense. The cocktail of chemo was more complex and stronger, so the side effects hit him harder. I had a feeling we were about to experience the rough road that had been described by seasoned veterans last fall when we first began. I braced myself.

But we were halfway done with the week, which was something to celebrate!

Ryder slept a lot, ate a little, and took in what fresh air he could. He stayed on a strict schedule with the anti-nausea meds this time, and they were working.

Missing My Family

It was hard to be disconnected from my other two children. I knew they needed me, though they seemed to be enjoying their independence and lack of supervision. I was grateful we had such a depth of community and that I could trust Reed would be looked after even when I couldn't see him. He spent a lot of time with his theater and choir pals, who had become his second family.

As a college sophomore, Woody was juggling the pursuit of his lifelong dreams with being so far away from what was happening with his older brother. He only shared his challenges at college with me, but I knew there had to be fears and conflicts he was keeping from me.

A hovering mom was the last thing either of them needed, but I longed to know what was going on in their hearts. I longed to tell them what was going on in mine.

Meanwhile, Chris was working, happily but nonstop. He did spend late nights at the hospital after I went home to bed, which helped. We were like ships passing in the night. We each knew the other was there somewhere, but our paths rarely crossed. Just when communication could have been our bedrock, we couldn't find the time to talk.

Not that he was the most open communicator. I knew this about him, but it was harder than ever to accept it. When I was especially frustrated, I had to remind myself what Chris' work brought to our table: magic, a comfortable life, and a content daddy.

NIKKI

Founding Member of Ryder's Band

Ryder had a special light about him. Whether he was talking about Bear (one of the dopest dogs I have ever met), imagining the future, or playing guitar, there was always a fire behind his eyes. And that was something really cool about being around Ryder. He was always excited about something.

I'll never forget that fire the last day I saw him. It was one of the first times I'd seen him since the cancer was cleared, and it was shortly after seeing Edward Sharpe and the Magnetic Zeros, his favorite band. He talked about the concert as he threw the frisbee in and out of the pool for the dogs. His hair was growing back fuzzier and blonder than ever. He glowed.

I was with an actor friend that day who had never met Ryder. I could tell he was transfixed. So transfixed that we were losing light for shooting at a location in the mountains that Ryder offered to show us. Cut to an hour later, and we were finally walking down the trail with snacks, gear, and camera in hand. About 45 minutes later, my friend asked Ryder, "Hey man, how much further until we get to this river, you think?"

"Oh, it's just around the corner."

Another 45 minutes later there was still no sign of the river. Since we were competing with daylight, we had to stop and set up. I thought at that point Ryder would be slightly bummed and turn back, but no. He was absolutely carefree and said with a wide smile that he was going to keep walking and catch the sunset. He strode out of sight, like a legend straight out of a movie.

QUIET DAYS

Ryder spent many more days moving from bed to couch and back again. He woke up in a sweat every hour during the night with anxious dreams, which left him exhausted. But on the flip side, that also meant he was awake to take his anti-nausea meds.

Despite all of this, Ryder maintained his heroic spirit. *"No victims allowed,"* he'd say. He was open to the treatment, and he accepted it gratefully and with patience. He seemed to have a grasp of the big picture. This eased his mental and emotional state, even though he said he was *"sick and tired of being sick and tired."*

While Ryder would demand the ultimate in nutritious fare from me, he'd waltz into the house with a bag from his favorite fast-food joint.

When he didn't feel like leaving the house, he dozed in front of endless soccer games on TV. Ryder wasn't up to reading even the most inspirational books, and the guitar stood patiently in the corner, waiting.

The doctor soon gave us great news on his progress and a prescription to help Ryder sleep. We took a very short walk later that day, hoping it would relieve some of the stressful dreams and help him get a good night's rest.

Before bed, we watched Survivor. Yes, indeed!

Talking Travel

Ryder found a world music class in Bali that summer that he wanted to attend. He needed something to anticipate. It was too early to plan, but I told him we'd see.

At the same time, I was considering chaperoning Reed's choir tour down the Danube between Ryder's third and fourth rounds of treatment.

Wherever I would feel the least guilt was where I would be. Guilt for not being at Ryder's beck and call during the fight for his life, or guilt for missing what I knew would be the highlight of Reed's young life? It seemed irreconcilable at the time, so I waited for the answer to come.

Time with Reed was moving up on my priority list. He clearly needed my attention, and I knew some of his acting out was due to an emptiness between us. He relished his independence but still needed me for support. A kid just needs to know his mom is there, even if she's simply a boundary to push away. This inner conflict made him angry—at me.

I couldn't say what I would do yet, but both boys said they would understand whatever I decided. If Ryder was doing as well during the next round, I could comfortably leave him in my mother's and sister's capable care.

CHRIS

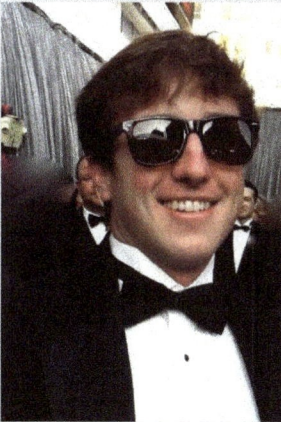

In 2011, Ryder and I got to go to the Oscars together. Whenever I took anyone else, they just wanted to watch the show. Not so with Ryder.

As soon as we arrived, he did a shout-out to Emma Stone, yelling, *"I want to marry you!"* Then he invited her to his show the following week.

Once we were seated and the program began, Ryder took off. I kept texting him as one hour went by…then two hours…"Where are you? What's going on?" And he would text back, *"I'm just hanging out with (this or that celebrity.)"* He spent the whole night schmoozing with people.

I thought, "Oh, shit! He's annoying some film producer, trying to get one of his songs in their film. Or he's getting drunk at the bar with all the losing actors who were drowning their sorrows.

Or worse yet, he's cornered Emma Stone somewhere and is passionately singing her one of his love songs."

About three hours later, just before they announced the Best Picture winner, Ryder finally made it back to his seat. He was grinning from ear to ear, a signal to me that there had to be a really good story.

When we got home, he told Shelley about all the connections he'd made. And yes, he did get a producer's contact information. But his proudest moment was his interaction with a girl he'd met who was running the elevator. He said he'd gotten her number and they'd kissed. Shelley was floored. "Say what? You picked someone up in the elevator at the Oscars?!"

He looked like a million bucks in his tuxedo and shades; he was putting himself out there and having a ball. It was so much fun to see. I knew that night that Ryder was no longer the quiet and reserved young boy I used to know. He was now a confident and fearless young man, ready to take on the world.

The girl did surface later. After he passed, somebody wrote about this story on his Facebook page, and she commented, "I'm the girl in the elevator."

Time Together

Ryder and I worked our way through Game of Thrones, a thrilling, yet sometimes racy, diversion. I think Ryder got a kick out of the fact that I could (barely) tolerate the sex and violence. But it was time with my grown son, so it was worth the effort. We watched as many episodes as his stamina would allow, often three or four in a sitting.

Watching TV eventually got tiresome, so one Sunday, Chris offered to drive Ryder to the beach. He jumped at the chance. Our house is about an hour from the coast, so this would be a rare treat for them both.

Being beach babies at heart, Chris knew the ocean waves and gentle breeze would provide a calming, nurturing, and healing environment for them both.

They drove out to one of their favorite spots, Zuma beach, just north of Malibu. They had their trunks on and were packed with towels, snacks, and beach chairs, all ready for a fantastic few hours.

As they parked, Chris said they noticed the beach was empty. "Wow, lucky us," they thought. "We've got the place to ourselves!"

Then they got out of the car. The wind slammed into them, almost knocking them off their feet. This was not what they expected, but they were determined to make the best of it. They trudged through the sand, finally planting their chairs close to the water.

Unfortunately, body surfing was out of the question since the waves were too choppy.

The sun was still shining, but because of the wind, the temperature was easily 20 to 30 degrees cooler than at home. So they bundled up in their sweatshirts and hunkered down into their chairs like a couple of turtles pulling their heads back into their shells.

Chris was trying to do a crossword puzzle, and Ryder was trying to read as the wind blew stronger and stronger, thrashing their faces with stinging sand. But nothing was going to stop them from having fantastic father/son bonding time.

They lasted 30 minutes, max, and then raced back to the car. They laughed all the way home and blew happily in the door long before I expected them.

While they were gone, I scheduled family massages for the next day as a surprise. This was a new experience for Reed, and he was skeptical. I had to insist, assuring him he would thank me when it was over. Massages required Chris and me to let go, which was a rarity these days, and who knew what goodness Reed would get out of it. Ryder relished the idea.

When it was over, there was a palpable sense of bonding among the four of us. As we sat in the glow of our relaxation, Reed asked, "When can we do that again, Mom?"

A few days later, Reed got sick with the flu. Had we forgotten to get him a shot? Possibly.

While I picked at the scab on my guilt, the brothers were sharing the bucket...how sweet.

Fleeting Serenity

Just when I was starting to relax, Ryder thought camping sounded like a good idea. Really?

After a hearty lunch, he packed the car with extra sleeping bags and a full cooler and then set out to pick up friends for the five-hour drive to Big Sur. One of the most iconic scenes on the California coast, it offers campgrounds perched atop the cliffs, sea lions lounging on the sand below, and stunning sunsets over the ocean. I couldn't stand in the way of that!

And then, like a boomerang, Ryder returned 30 minutes later to just *"chill"* and leave in the morning. Though he was reluctant to admit it, he just didn't have the energy for the trip quite yet. I was SO relieved! The relief only lasted a day, though, because he was off and running the next morning.

The ups and downs just never stopped.

Countdown to Round Three

After he returned from his camping trip, Ryder and I got lunch at our favorite Mediterranean restaurant. They serve healthy food, so we always left feeling good, and as Ryder said, *"without guilt."* Then we went home to watch a few more Game of Thrones episodes.

That night, I started to pack for the European trip with Reed. I had made my decision. Reed needed me more. My mom and sister would take care of Ryder at home between treatments while I was gone. I wanted so much to have this time with Reed. He'd taken the back seat for months now, and we both needed this shared adventure.

IMPATIENCE MEETS NAUSEA

The Monday morning check-in started with the same torturous chair in Ryder's room. It was too firm, didn't recline, and apparently wasn't made to fit an actual body. Especially for the 10 hours I spent in it each day.

The view this time was nicer, though. We could look out over the campus grounds filled with trees and vast expanses of green grass.

And his lab numbers were very, very good!

So two steps forward and one inconvenience. Well, make that two inconveniences. By late afternoon, they still couldn't get Ryder's IV hooked up. His veins weren't cooperating. He didn't complain, but we all know how needles feel. After two strikes, they had to fetch the tiny needle specialist.

After this week, I'd be home with Ryder for another four days before I left for my trip with Reed, and I was glad for it. I imagined this round's recovery would be tougher since Ryder never really regained his stamina after the last round. He had spurts of energy followed by lots of horizontal time.

AUNT SHANLEY

Ryder had a big heart for such a young man. He was a great toddler and little boy with a mischievous smile and a kind and loving nature. I can't help but think of an adorable picture I have with Ryder and my son, RJ, his cousin. The two of them had goofy little grins on their faces and were holding plastic water guns. I laugh when I think of this because Shelley did not want Ryder to have toy guns. But she finally gave in when Ryder was so desperate that he made his toast into the shape of a gun.

Countdown to Friday

As my departure date neared, it occurred to me that the specific errands Ryder asked of me, then rejected, might have been an unconscious test of *"Do you love me enough to…"* along with a message of *"Nothing you do will make me feel better."* I heard him loud and clear. But I would never stop trying.

So I fetched smoothies, brought homemade meals to his hospital room, and prepped Grandma Dot and Aunt Leslie on every detail of home care (basically, cater to his every whim). Distract him if you can. Have FUN! I knew they would.

Before leaving the hospital that week, Ryder gave the doctor an earful in his firm but gentle voice. He didn't want to come back for his next, and hopefully last, round. I couldn't blame him. This. Was. Hard. He said he'd rather be at home barfing than here. No needles, free reign to step outside, his choice of music and videos. No interruptions. NO BEEPING.

The doctor didn't argue Ryder's point. He treated him with compassion and understanding, gave gentle directions, told Ryder the benefits of the full treatment, and then left quietly. I saw that for what it was. The doctor wasn't going to take up arms, but he also wasn't going to budge.

I spent more time sitting in the courtyard under the trees, by the fountains, beside the fish tank, in the piano atrium or the meditation room with the stained glass. But just after I returned that day, the doctor came in and looked at me as if to say, "You're here? Again? Still?" I assured him I was not there to watchdog the staff. They were so good on both a personal and professional level.

And I wouldn't forget the night Ryder said, *"Everything went to hell when you left, Mom."* I had left early, before a visitor arrived and stayed too long. It was another reason for me to be there. I could have run interference and said it was time for Ryder to sleep. Something. Anything. He felt helpless, and he didn't know how to set boundaries with someone who'd made the effort to come.

So yes, I was still there.

Grandma Dot had been at home with Reed all week. This was a huge relief for me, but Chris was starting to show some cracks.

Work was proceeding at break-neck speed, and his little sister had just been through hip surgery (a big deal for Mary, who is overweight and has Down syndrome). Chris never complained, but that night he said his heart broke every day for Ryder. This was the first I'd heard from him about how he was feeling. While I wore my heart on my sleeve, he was anything but demonstrative. With that one comment, I knew he understood what I was experiencing, and I felt his support.

Chris didn't talk about his heartache to me, perhaps out of compassion for what he knew I was going through. It was his character to spare me.

Though we may never know what small comfort Ryder got when he opened his eyes to see one of us, we thought it was worth it to be there for whatever comfort it did bring.

It Ain't "The Care Bears Get Chemo"

There was nothing light and airy about these times. It was grueling. As the week wore on, Ryder became more and more irritable. I was holding my breath, hoping to just get through it and be back home.

I could soldier on as long as he was cooperating, but his outburst on the last day in the hospital brought me to tears.

He threatened not to come back, saying, *"You don't know what this FEELS like. YOU aren't going through it. YOU get to go home."*

He was right. I was able to go home, to move freely in the world. But even though I wasn't hooked up, cooped up, poked and prodded, I was going through my own version of hell watching it all.

I blocked the idea that this treatment might be a futile exercise and that the cancer might be fatal, after all. I believed in his doctor, in the confidence he exuded. I could not imagine life without my first-born boy. So I just didn't let myself entertain those thoughts.

I could bear anything as long as Ryder did this, fully and completely. He was so close. After this treatment, he'd have a two-week break. Then just five more days of treatment. To trade five days of discomfort for a chance at life seemed like a no-brainer to me. For better odds at never having to do this again, all the pain and hassle seemed worth it. When he made threats to leave like that I couldn't help but feel his perspective got lost. Wasn't it worth the fight to be alive?

He put a time limit on it. *"Out by 3:00 p.m. or I'm ripping these tubes out and never coming back."*

I didn't blame him for feeling that way, but he was trying my patience.

That morning, he dragged his feet getting out of the house, procrastinating, finding any distraction to delay our departure.

"They never see me on time anyway," Ryder said.

Never mind that he was the first appointment of the day, and they were waiting for him. Forget he'd been told at the outset that the earlier he got to the lab, the sooner he could start his treatment.

So we got to the lab 30 minutes late, and he was in line behind about eight to 10 people. If we showed up to our appointment late, that didn't mean our day would be delayed by just 30 minutes. It meant all the people ahead of us got their potions concocted before we did, which took time. Hours in this case.

We were stuck waiting in line in a tiny room with a dozen other people. I let the circumstances speak for themselves with my silence.

For the entire week, both day- and night-time staff scrambled to do everything they could to make up that time. They cajoled the pharmacy and doubled up his infusions, doing everything they could to speed up the process. Still, he'd be lucky to get out by 6:00 p.m. on Friday.

What I couldn't abide was blaming the nurses. He grumbled about their performance. Why couldn't they just get it started? I was seething. The whole delay pointed to Ryder, but stating the obvious would just make the situation worse, so I bit my tongue. Again.

Could it be that he had just lost it by this point in the week? Most certainly. The next day, Friday, he would be released, and he knew it wouldn't be early due to his own choices.

AUNT LESLIE

Shelley's Sister

On Ryder's sixth birthday, we had planned our first unchaperoned adventure—just the two of us. Even though we were going to SeaWorld, I told him we had to stop at a toy store on the way to get some items I needed for an art project.

When we got there, Ryder made a beeline for the dinosaurs. Like a lot of kids who grew up watching Jurassic Park, he had an impressive, almost encyclopedic knowledge of dinosaurs.

He showed me what would have been the crown jewel of his collection: T-Rex. He said he really, really wanted this for his birthday. I said, "OK Ryder, if that's what you really want, that's what I want you to have. But if we buy T-Rex, we'll just go back home and go to SeaWorld another day."

He said, *"I want to go to SeaWorld."* He was very definite about it. I complimented him on what a mature decision that was, and we headed out to the car.

He was quiet for a couple of minutes, then he smiled at me as bright as could be and said, *"Well, you know why I said that? Because Christmas is coming up. You can buy me that T-Rex for Christmas!"*

I was so proud of him at that moment because he was learning to work the angles, and he never really stopped. That was my boy.

The Real Deal

So this was cancer. The real deal. It had really set in.

His favorite nurse was there on his last day of treatment that week, which was a good thing for us all. I had a moment to speak to her in the hall, and I mentioned his protests about another round of chemo. He said he was not coming back, which shook me to my core. I could only hope he'd settle down and comply. I was counting on it. He'd been this cranky before and had come through with calm and grace. We would just have to wait and see.

He had already told his nurse he wasn't returning. Everyone within a 10-mile radius understood that he felt this way by the end of the week.

"Of course we want to see him again, and not just here—on stage somewhere," the nurse said, tearing up.

No wonder she cried. She got it. She'd had patients refuse treatment. She'd seen people die because of bad choices. She didn't want the same for Ryder.

Ah, Home at Last

He was glad to be home and stopped talking about refusing treatment. I held my breath and said little. I certainly wasn't going to argue the point because that would just make him more resolute. I made myself scarce, until he needed me.

Ryder woke up in the middle of the night drenched in sweat with stressful dreams. The next morning, he got into the pool, dreamed of his favorite Hawaiian beaches, and rested in the hammock. It wiped him out. He rotated from the bed to the couch for the rest of the day.

Ryder was reluctant to take the anti-nausea meds—mostly because they caused the bad dreams—and he paid the price. The barf bucket was always within reach.

I got a massage to repair my back after a long day in the dreaded hospital chair and then finished packing. I thought it would be a nice break for Ryder to have "Cancer Mom" gone for a while. Europe would be a shot in the arm for me, and Reed was so excited he was bubbling.

Ryder felt much better, although he was still rather housebound by the time I was supposed to leave. I felt good leaving him with my sister and mother because I knew they'd keep him occupied. I would know he was really feeling good when he got the guitar out again and continued to bring his gift to the world.

Keepin' On

After months of indecision, Reed and I went off with an "au revoir!"

Europe was a trial. Being separated from Ryder was a shock to my soul, but the music the students made was glorious. They sang acapella in small churches and grand cathedrals along the banks of the Danube. The settings were centuries old and breathtaking. One hundred students from our high school blended their voices to create a heavenly sound which brought parents and local spectators to tears. The weather outside was rainy and gray, but the venues and the students' faces brought color to the scene.

I found myself smiling a lot and tearing up often. I couldn't be sure if it was the music or what I was going through at home that made them flow. Both, I guess.

There were rewards, to be sure: a sweet glance from Reed across the dining room, a quick whisper about the dessert he thought I'd like, a tearful hug at the end of a concert.

"I love you so much, Mom," he said on a number of occasions.

Any doubt I had about being there melted away. This was where I needed to be. Where I wanted to be.

In my room at night, I did my silent connecting with Ryder. I let him be, with no phone calls, but my heart was definitely in two places.

UNCLE DON

When Aunt Flo and I were visiting, we'd sleep in Ryder's bed. He always came in and gave me a kiss goodnight...because that is what you do in that room at night. You tuck people in with love. I'll never forget that.

Returning to Silence

After 10 days in gray, wintry Europe, it felt good to return to Southern California's sunshine and spring colors. However, I learned Ryder had not picked up the guitar since Reed and I left. That spoke volumes about his state of being.

Check-in for the final week of inpatient treatment would come the morning following our return. I knew this one would be tough.

Ryder was on time checking into the cancer center, but there was no joy in Mudville that day. He was hoping for rain all week. Rain and sleep. He asked about sedatives, and I didn't blame him. But the doctor just chuckled.

We talked about tricks to pass the time:

- Watching movies
- Pretending that he had several more rounds, instead of just this one (please!)
- Looking forward to concerts and trips
- Considering this threshold the doorway to a new life

Still, those games wouldn't erase the imminent discomfort he knew all too well. He didn't even bring his guitar this week. I hoped he'd sleep. I intended to be there all day, every day, unless it seemed to tire him. Chris would continue to go in at night, mostly just to sit.

Many times, Ryder would just be so tired, he'd be sleeping when Chris got there. Or he'd seem like he was asleep. One night, Chris got up very quietly and tiptoed to the door.

"You don't have to leave," Ryder said.

"Oh, you're awake," Chris said.

"Yeah."

Chris sat back down. Ryder still didn't talk to him. He just wanted him to be there. That's all. It was a sweet thing, and it made Chris feel that the time he spent at the hospital at night was well worth it.

RYDER

If a man feels only goodness, does he really know how to feel?

Not completely, because feeling the hurt is what helps open a mind;
looking above for a power divine.

His insides are twisted, into knots they get tied,
as he floats ever onward, awaiting a sign.

Some shiver of soul, so great that he knows,
no matter the course, he is never alone.

A Hitch in Our Git Along

Ryder was pale and slightly green when I returned on Sunday. This may have been too gradual a change for anyone who was with him daily to notice, but it struck me the minute I laid eyes on him.

The lab reports we got at check-in that Monday morning showed Ryder was very anemic. This explained why he was still taking naps the whole time I was in Europe.

While I was helping Ryder get settled in for the week, he shared a new favorite band with me. I was immediately taken with Alex Ebert's Edward Sharpe and the Magnetic Zeros (ESMZ), seeing the same things Ryder did: the genuine heart, the gratitude for life, and the humility of the entire band.

ESMZ—more than any other band—had become a staple in his days. Ryder related to Alex's return from darker days, even a brush with death. It made Alex human and his celebration of life more authentic. Ryder was determined to beat the monster inside him, and Alex was an example of what could be.

By early afternoon, I gave in to my jet lag and went home for a short nap. Ryder was getting grumpy by then, and I thought some rest might help him, too. But at 4:00 p.m., he called me ranting that chemo hadn't started yet because he needed a blood transfusion.

The first transfusion took five hours. This put him seriously behind on his Friday checkout, and that was his greatest concern. He threatened to walk out the door on Friday, no matter what.

LEXI

Friend from Musicians Institute

Ryder and I were both aspiring singer/songwriters, which is how we met. Our first conversation was shortly after he had finished chemotherapy when he told me how his music and his mom had saved him. We spent hours jamming/writing together, and I'll never forget how stubborn he was or how much joy he got out of life.

The Race Was On

The lab results came in, and Ryder's numbers were within their target range, so this final round was for "insurance," quoting the doctor. I never told Ryder that. My fingers were crossed.

The nurse assured him they could get him out Friday. With little or no break in the chemo, they thought they'd be able to catch up. But no doubt it would be harder on him. He asked Chris to spend the night on Friday so he could leave as soon as it was finished. We all felt hopeful.

As the days wore on, Ryder became more passive with no energy left to fight. My heart ached for him. Every minute of every day, I longed for a smile and fervently prayed that this would be the last of it. Though he knew others had endured more, this was the toughest challenge of his young life, and it had to be enough.

I was near tears for days because I saw the end of treatment coming. Please, God, let this be the end.

Perky Thursday

What? He took a shower! This was the first one since he checked in on Monday. Normally fastidious about his hygiene, it struck me hard that he hadn't bothered. He looked disheveled. It was a clear indicator of his state of mind during that long last week of treatment. He was dragging but enthusiastic about going home the next day for what we hoped would be the last time.

Counting the hours to Friday, he hooked up his computer and fired up his phone. He felt lousy enough that I knew he wouldn't be making any plans for Friday night, but he was reconnecting with friends, hoping to get together in the following days.

The staff was tripping over themselves to make him comfortable. He said it was only the day team that gave such great care, but Chris had been there the night before and said they were sweet. I knew the subtext was, *"Nothing can make this better."*

Oh well, I was sure the shower helped. Sheesh.

TGIF!

It was a long day, but things went smoothly enough. Anyone who peeked in his door heard he wanted out and *"The sooner, the better."* Man, were they scrambling! I truly believe the whole staff did their utmost to meet his schedule. Not that we had a train to catch, but the sun was not coming up on Ryder's bed at the cancer center the next day. No sir.

Finally, his robot beeped, signaling the end of treatment. The aide poked her head in, and someone parked a wheelchair just outside his room. We were homeward bound!

I hated to count my chickens. We had celebrated before, but I simply had to be grateful this part was over. There would surely be more to come in the form of scans, blood tests, and follow-up appointments. But there was time to talk about that later

As we drove away from the cancer center, he said, *"I am SO glad to be getting away from this PLACE. There are just no words to describe this feeling. Of FINALLY going home. Of being done."*

Whispering

Could this really be over? We had yet to get his markers, but Ryder felt it was. He knew it wasn't really over last November, but he felt it was now. He'd have to be careful not to get an infection since his blood counts were low, but every step toward feeling better held promise.

He said he felt like dancing. His bare feet on the grass brought a smile. Oh, what a treasure, that smile!

The doctor told us we would have to come back in a month for a checkup. Ryder would get scans and blood tests a week before that. By then he would have gone up north for a concert, and his hair would have started to grow back. We planned a concert and party in the back yard for late May to celebrate. We wanted to invite everyone who'd supported us through this journey.

Our world had stopped spinning the previous September, and we were oh-so-ready to start moving on.

AUNT BARB

Having heard Ryder perform at a family reunion, we were inspired to ask him to play when I got remarried. We asked if he knew "In My Life" by the Beatles. Not only did he know the song, but he was excited to have Woody harmonize with him. They showed up in coordinating shirts and ties, and of course, Ryder was in his signature flip-flops. He assured me, though, that these were his dress flip-flops.

The Aftermath

For nine months, I'd lived on the verge of tears. Of pent-up stress. Of being poised for anything, ever on guard, holding my breath and waiting.

Though the waiting wasn't over, there was no sense putting life on hold any longer. The jewelry business beckoned, but my energy was low, and I didn't have much direction. I wandered the house, rudderless, randomly picking up the pieces. It appeared my focus and drive would take some time to return.

Meanwhile, Ryder had been shot out of a cannon. He'd have an up day where he did too much, then a down day to recover. He spent a lot of time in the pool because exercise helped with sleep more than any pill.

The slow days made him irritable as his mind was ready to go, go, go!

His appetite came back in full force, then not so much. He was still riding a wave.

I was beginning to believe his condition of the past few weeks had been tied to a deep-seated dread, a depression of sorts. Even if it was just a result of his body feeling lousy, at least that cloud had lifted.

He seemed to need to separate from me, the "Cancer Mom." We talked about that, bringing it to consciousness.

One day, I caught him at the kitchen island, making himself something to eat. I knew I had a captive audience for a few minutes.

"I am not the disease. I didn't bring it with me," I said. The cancer was a touchy subject, and I didn't know what to expect in response. Surprisingly, Ryder was open to a discussion.

"I know, Mom. I just want to put this all behind me. Everything about home reminds me of the cancer. I just need to forget. I have to get out of here, sometimes."

Though he denied blaming me for anything that had occurred over the last nine months, I still felt like he wanted to run from me.

The distance he was trying to establish hurt. We had been through something so profound together, and I yearned for that closeness to continue. I wanted to celebrate together. I knew I was inextricably connected to his cancer experience, and it wasn't anything I could shake. All I could do was bring my feelings into the light.

If he could have moved out, he would have then. But he was a student with no job, and he only had his car for brief escapes.

But still, he wanted to forget, and I was a constant reminder.

Ryder wanted to take the wheel, but I had driven this whole process. I was accustomed to leading the charge, and I was having a hard time letting go. Well, it was natural, I guess, to throw the baby out with the bath water. And I was that baby.

Ryder Takes the Wheel

Two days after being released, Ryder decided to go hiking.

Ok, I thought, it's rattlesnake weather. Besides that, he was still very pale.

I served up some beets, berries, carrots, cucumber, coconut water, ginger, and ice, which he chased with a fistful of supplements. And I prayed. The hike wiped him out, but fortunately he was with a good friend and came home safely. And I hadn't mentioned the snakes. Mommy was growing!

As part of rebuilding his life, Ryder drove himself to the hospital for a routine checkup. The results of prior blood work were in, and the numbers were alarming. The doctor liked platelets to be at 100,000 during chemo, and his were at 6,000! His hemoglobin was down to 6.3, but 10 is where it should have been.

This explained why he was bruised and had a bloody nose the night before. Ryder was starting to bleed spontaneously, which is why Dr. Quinn told him he would need three units of blood and one or two units of platelets immediately. He'd have to be there for at least eight hours.

Ryder called to tell me the news, insisting he'd be fine and that no one needed to come to the hospital. I decided to listen to him and stay at home. Little did I know, he was hatching a plan.

I thought he was still at the hospital when the nurse called. They had been paging Ryder and searching everywhere for him. She was clearly alarmed.

Ryder had left the hospital against medical advice! The nurse said she didn't want him to "bleed out." I was beside myself.

I called out for help, writing a quick post on CaringBridge.org, my communication link to all our friends and family. That was all it took. Calls and visitors came flooding in.

I couldn't reach Chris by phone, which added to my growing panic. I called the wife of a friend at Disney, whose husband let Chris know we needed him.

My sister-in-law went to track Ryder down with me, hoping he was still on the hospital grounds.

About a half hour after the nurse's call, he showed up at home, self-satisfied. He explained that he just didn't want another IV and didn't believe this was *"that big of a deal."* Then he took up his position on the couch and dialed up a soccer game.

Chris came home early and begged Ryder to go to the hospital, saying, "I never ask anything of you." I stood by, helplessly crying.

Our doctor and nurse friends showed up by phone or in person to cajole him.

He refused treatment. He said he was not prepared for an IV that day. He said he would do it the next week if he still needed it.

All of these things added up to major concerns for the doctors.

This was more immediately life-threatening than the cancer was. He could bleed to death just lying on the couch. Why I couldn't get the urgency of this through to him was putting me on the brink of hysteria. I was broken.

AMY

Family Friend

Early in 2013, my friend had a dream that my sister and I were mourning a young man while we were at a wedding. The letters "RB" were part of the dream, and though Ryder was a good friend, the idea that it could be him never crossed our minds. Then Ryder passed suddenly, and his service was held on the very day our other sister was getting married.

Our Army

The responses to my SOS came flooding in.

A close friend of mine called him with a doctor's warning that a stroke and blindness were very possible.

Woody called him, concerned.

Aunt Leslie got him to agree to go in the next day.

Luisa closed the shop early and made dinner for us. He needed to eat. She provided a distraction so he didn't feel ambushed by his parents.

Another friend brought dinner and encouraging words. We had plenty to eat that night, and it was a good thing because the house was full.

A nurse friend came over for a serious talk. Her good counsel was, "You needed to be in control. You did that. Now go do what you need to do."

Someone suggested a spiritual advisor come by the next day. I jumped on it.

Uncle Doug did everything Reed needed, handling his backpack, food, and transportation to rehearsal.

Countless people emailed.

We had offers to donate blood.

What would I have done without our friends? My army.

Not So Fast, Sir

Together, all of this concern convinced Ryder to go back to the hospital but on his terms. He finally went in that night, but not until the soccer game was over.

By 7:00 a.m., they were still calling for one more unit each of blood and platelets. All told, they gave him four units of blood and two units of platelets. Then they decided to keep him overnight.

Ryder was resigned. No more protests. The doctor and head nurse impressed on him the seriousness of his condition. They explained what "bleed out" meant. We had covered this at home, but it finally sank in coming from the doctor.

Home

When Ryder was released at 12:30 p.m. the next day, I took him out for some hearty burgers at his favorite steak house. His temperament had mellowed. He was happy to be out, as if it had been no big deal.

We chatted about anything but what we'd just been through. I was distraught, but I hid it. No sense beating a dead horse. And Ryder was triumphant, so I went with that.

His color was better, but it still wasn't great. They wanted to see him back in a few days. There was still a chance that he would need more blood and platelets.

For now, we had dodged another bullet!

JENNY

Ryder's Friend

One time after hanging out, Ryder offered to give me a ride home. Taking the freeway south would have gotten us there in no time. Instead, we took what he called, *"the long way,"* which added at least 10 more minutes. He told me he preferred this route because it had winding roads lined with beautiful trees. This experience has always stuck with me because it reminds me of how Ryder enriched our lives by showing us how to love, enjoy life, spend more time with those we care about, and do the things that make us happy.

Hurry Up, Monday

Ryder's pattern since his release from the hospital was waking up early then going back to sleep on the couch. He developed a persistent cough. We were two weeks out from his last treatment. Normally, he would have rebounded by now, but he was only up for about one outing per day. His color still wasn't good. His complexion was pale and a little greenish, and the place on his arm where the last needle went in days ago still looked fresh, red, and angry.

He was scheduled for CT scans before his next appointment the following Monday. Dr. Quinn also said he would need another infusion of blood. I tried to gently prepare Ryder so he would cooperate. Breaking the news, I slipped it into an easy conversation. He was amenable, so there was nothing more to be said.

Believe me, I would do the driving this time.

But before the Monday appointment, we decided he needed to go back to the hospital. He had developed black circles under his eyes and lost the color in his lips. When we got there, they were ready and waiting for him. In that light, I noticed more bruising on his arms and legs. His whole body was pale and greenish. The doctor also discovered signs of a nosebleed.

Ryder was mentally prepared for an admission, but the test results were good enough to send him home. The doctor said one of the numbers indicated his bone marrow was actively producing blood cells.

Though we didn't feel we were quite at the celebration point, we both felt giddy!

By the time of his appointment the following week, we hoped we would learn he was continuing to head in the right direction.

Meanwhile, I tried to catch up on life. Reed had his first solo choral performance, I had some jewelry orders to finish up, a photo album of Reed's Europe trip to send to print, and Woody would soon return from Michigan.

Both Reed and Woody required attention, but Reed was more demonstrative. "I neeeeed you to bring dinner for the cast!" Woody was a whirlwind of activities he wanted to share with me. This left no time for doting on Ryder or taking time for myself. I had to get my showers in at dawn or not until late in the day. The dogs needed to be walked. Fortunately, Chris was also an early riser, so we got a little time together before he left for work.

Looking Forward

We were changing gears. I was sitting in neutral, rolling slowly downhill with one foot poised over the brake. Ryder was inching forward, though his mind raced ahead.

He prioritized and made lists with optimism and caution. His summer plans included work and travel and then eventually going back to school in the fall. We still had to wait a couple of weeks for the "all clear." We knew there were no guarantees, but we had to proceed "as if."

SALLY

College Counselor

Reference Letter for Bali Study Abroad Music Program

Ryder Buck is a calm, self-assured, gracious young adult. He is accepting of the differences in people; in fact, he celebrates the wisdom and consciousness that his relationships with a diverse group of friends brings. He comes across as a person with "inner peace."

Ryder is well suited for intensive study. He will bring the self-discipline necessary for personal success to this program; he will have every intention to learn as much as he can and derive optimal benefit from this study abroad experience. He wants to know how things work together and will be an efficient student and an effective communicator. Ryder will fit beautifully with your program. He has an open mind and is eager to learn and grow.

Comfortable with himself and around others, Ryder has the ability to make people feel good when they are around him (I write this even though I firmly believe that no one can make anyone else feel a certain way.) He is inquisitive, loves to learn, and can teach himself almost anything he puts his mind to. He loves to share, teach, and entertain. I am convinced that the guitar has become an actual body part— Ryder composes, writes lyrics, and performs with a grace and effortlessness that draws others to him for "more!" He is extremely entertaining but serious when he needs to be. I believe he adds color, life, and love to whatever he touches.

Ryder Buck knows no limits. The combination of energy, tenacity, and intellectual curiosity will make him a valuable addition to your program. And you won't meet a nicer guy!

WAITING TO BREATHE

A few weeks after his final treatment, Ryder began feeling better. He was in and out most days, mostly out. When he'd head out the door at midnight, I'd hear my grandmother's voice in my head from when I was 18. "Oh, don't go out now. I will worry." I dismissed her with a laugh and a wave of my hand. I think I even said something like, "That would be your problem." So I bit my tongue with Ryder.

Ah, karma. And I had Reed, lest I ever forgot. He now had his license and could drive himself to water polo practice at 6:30 a.m. That was a relief for the rest of us, though we still had to get him out of bed.

I got a few golden moments with Ryder when his social life and music-making weren't pulling him away. Our favorite thing to do was watch Survivor on CBS. It was where the clock stopped, and we set everything else aside.

I admit I'm a sucker for the show, but what I was really hankering for was some quality time with my son. We each cheered for our favorite player. This fun little competition was a needed change from our mother-son dynamics of the past months. Plus, studying the psychology of the game made for rich conversations. Ryder's intuition was uncanny.

Low Hanging Fog

When I finally had time to reflect on the recent choir trip, I realized that there must be an underlying pall to my life. I had offered to assemble a photo album of the trip and collect and place everyone's orders for prints. I would normally have done this immediately after the trip, but I couldn't get started until things settled down with Ryder. Even then, I was dragging my heels.

Memories of the trip were great. Though photos of the scenery were mostly gray, they had a beauty of their own. The faces of the kids were bright, as colorful as the breathtaking interiors of the cathedrals where they sang. I enjoyed every moment with them, including the midnight games of hide-and-seek, which they always won. It made me smile to remember it.

So why was I so relieved when it was over?

There was still so much I could do and had to do at home. Chris was working late nights and weekends. Time stretched out in front of me, and yet I wasn't motivated.

There WERE joyful moments. Reed's performances were delightful events, and I was proud of him. Woody completed his sophomore year with stellar reviews. I had so much to celebrate. And yet, I was still holding my breath.

MARKOS

Instructor at Musicians Institute

I had spent the better part of 20 years touring the world and making records. Musicians Institute offered me a teaching position, and I dove in with reckless enthusiasm. Ryder was one of my earliest students, and he was extraordinary. Years later, he remains one of my most impressive.

I remember helping Ryder refine a few of his standout originals, songs I believe still hold up as modern classics and likely could've become generation-defining radio singles.

Overall, he had a vision to merge what he called the "surf-chill" genre with postmodern blues. He was always willing to try any of my ideas, but he also had an innate courage of conviction and wasn't afraid to respectfully disagree when he felt the songs would be better as is.

I appreciated and admired his endearingly upbeat and positive can-do personality and his willingness to be pushed to achieve his maximum potential. His magnetic charisma, natural singing/guitar playing ability, and songwriting chops immediately evidenced that raw undefinable something that the industry refers to as "star power." Ryder effortlessly possessed that which cannot be taught. Every so often I've been fortunate enough to encounter artists who shared these rare traits. Most of them, unsurprisingly, became superstars.

It's always incomprehensible when a person dies young, but somehow the tragedy cuts even deeper when it happens to be an artist. You factor in the tremendous loss, not only to family and friends but also to culture and humanity. For these reasons, we not only mourn the loss of Ryder, the guy who personally touched our lives, but we also mourn the promise, joy, and love he would have undoubtedly brought to the world.

Some lights are so bright, they are destined to become stars. Perhaps, Ryder Buck has literally become one. After all, maybe that's what they mean by "star power." Shine on, Ryder Buck.

Was That the Sun Peeking Through?

The news we had been waiting for finally came at our last appointment for blood tests and CT scans. The CT scans were clear! His lymph nodes and lungs were all good. They were going to keep an eye on his liver function, but the end of this journey was in sight.

The doctor told Ryder not to go hiking in remote areas and get scratched up because his platelets and blood counts were still only teetering above transfusion level. And we'd have a precautionary appointment with his internist in a month. Still, his medical team was all smiles, and we genuinely felt like we could begin to dance our way back into life!

Ryder began to gear up for his comeback gig, which was set for three weeks later. It would be a fundraising concert to support Children's Hospital. We were proud of him for already wanting to give something back, and we hoped everyone who had been with us through this whole ordeal would come and help us celebrate.

In the meantime, he flew the coop to head up the coast for a concert and would be gone from Thursday through Sunday. His favorite band, ESMZ, was playing, and nothing could have kept him from going.

A Text

After 48 hours away from Ryder, I felt it was time for contact.

"You ok?"

"Yes. Today was life changing. So amazing. Tell you tomorrow."

That one exchange had me beaming. I couldn't wait to hear all about it. He SO needed this, and if he said the words *"life changing,"* I could only imagine it truly was.

When Ryder got home, he was absolutely gushing. He became a huge fan of the band when he discovered them during his first stay in the hospital. He felt an instant connection with their music and with the spirit of their leader, Alex Ebert. Seeing them in person moved him more than he could articulate. He sat right up front and marveled at their performance. He loved the poetry of their music and felt they told the most beautiful stories.

I was delighted for Ryder. He was living his life again with newfound depth and enthusiasm. It was beautiful to witness and warmed my heart. I could only imagine what this experience would mean for his own developing artistry.

EDDIE

Bandmate

I moved to LA from Texas to find my niche in the music industry. After six months, I hadn't played a lick of live music, and I was on the verge of going back home to my family, friends, and steady job.

Then I met Ryder.

He exuded warmth and a positive energy that I hadn't felt from anyone in LA. We talked extensively about our similar tastes in music. He told me that he was a songwriter and needed a second guitar player to cover a couple of shows. I couldn't have said "YES" fast enough!

Standing outside a bar one night, there was a street merchant selling roses. Ryder bought two and asked that the merchant give them to two pretty girls standing near us. Ryder didn't know them, but he had no problem spending money on those roses!

I said, "Dude, you shouldn't have done that. They're probably just going to take the roses and leave without even a 'thank you.'"

But Ryder wasn't expecting anything in return. He showed those girls a kindness just because. That was the very first of many "Ryder-isms" that completely changed my outlook on life.

Rough Days for Me

Now that I wasn't in full "Cancer Mom" armor, s*#% was starting to bubble up to the surface. I was glum, without direction, and distracted. Spending time with a few cherished friends helped, but then the void would return. I knew I would get my feet solidly under me again, but I had little patience for the antics that had previously gotten my attention around the house. I felt like I was alone in a crowd, head in a fog, and stubbornly so. It was weird.

Reed came just in time to redirect my focus. He could be counted on to jump in and require my attention, just when I needed to be left alone. His presence was never subtle, and as the third-born in our family, his job was clearly to climb the ranks.

After an evening of it, I went to bed early and woke up the next morning mentally packing for a solo trip to Hawaii. This dissolved into dreaming of a drive up the coast, which unfolded into a massage, errands, and lunch in Pasadena.

It was a good thing I hadn't gone far, though, as sometime early that afternoon Ryder found two lumps surrounded by reddish skin on his forearm. We called the doctor and he told us to keep a close eye on it.

Reed's prom was that same night. He said, "I need a shiny gold bow tie, Mom! And a matching pocket square, puhleeease!" Wait. Was this the same mom you were ready to devour two nights ago?

Ok, honey. Gold lamé, coming right up. I just needed to find my magic wand.

Grandma Dot had a choir recital at a local college with the boys' former high school teacher. Chris, Ryder, and Woody would be at the recital while I took prom pictures of Reed. This would be a mercifully quiet evening at home alone. Maybe I'd count my new gray hairs.

The Cough

Ryder's cough had become a character in our lives, and it was not going away.

We asked several doctors about it but got no answers. Everything about Ryder's condition was a source of concern. What might a cough indicate? Was it related to the cancer? Would it affect his overall health? Allergy meds did not relieve his symptoms. I believed antibiotics were long overdue, but Ryder was growing weary of medicine.

We eventually got an appointment with our internist. I hoped we could figure out how to quell the cough.

Finally

Ryder got the antibiotics he needed to fight a bacterial infection. While he was recovering, we found the right time and space to reflect on what we had been through together.

Even though this had been his cancer, it had affected our entire family and circle of friends, and Ryder and I had been joined at the hip through every moment of the experience. Some things were impossible to put into words, but we got enough of it out to allow each other to begin healing.

We talked about the pain of helplessness, both his and mine. I understood his sense of helplessness better than he related to mine, so this was a great place to begin.

He spoke of feeling trapped, of not being able to say, *"Go away. I want to be alone."*

Even as he needed me more than ever before, he also needed his independence. I told him parents would do anything to make their child better, including walk away, as long as they weren't allowing their child to do more harm to himself than he might realize.

He told me he felt humbled by the second cycle of treatment, which made him realize how attached he was to his hair and that he needed to let it go. His priorities started to shift. He realized the preciousness of time and the absolute need to surround himself with positive energy.

Again, we had to work through the fact that I didn't bring the disease with me, but rather, I needed to wear my superhero's cape into battle. At the time, he couldn't separate this out, but he eventually understood how those things had gotten blurred. Afterall, I had been there for every step of the battle. My presence was a constant reminder of what Ryder desperately wanted to put behind him. At the hospital, I could always go for a walk or into the lounge if I sensed he needed solitude. At home, it was impossible to be invisible or silent. I needed to talk about my experience, too.

After that conversation, I felt like we could move forward as partners with mutual respect for one another's healing processes. Few people realized I needed time to recover as well. Three months on a beach might have been a good start, but that wasn't going to happen. Instead, I learned to carve out little moments to consciously say "yes" to indulgences I might have otherwise skipped.

ASHLEY

Ryder's Friend

I had the amazing pleasure of meeting Ryder in the environment he loved—near the beach, at a gig, with family. His talent was obvious, along with his compassion, generosity, positivity, and heart. I will never forget how happy he looked up on stage.

Scattering

After a week, Ryder was free of the cough and off to La Jolla for a weekend with his old college roommate. Woody left for San Diego to see some plays. Reed was living at the high school's playhouse preparing for the opening of THE MUSIC MAN.

Thanks to a dear friend, I spent some time at a beach house up the coast. This was exactly what the doctor would have ordered.

RYDER

CaringBridge

First, I'd just like to say thank you. Thank you to anyone and everyone who has taken the time to check in, see how I was, pick up the phone, lend advice, click a heart, or send their love/positive energy. I wouldn't be feeling as good as I am now if it weren't for all of you amazing people who know me in one way or another. It blows me away to see just how many people out there knew about my situation and were pulling for my recovery since this whole whirlwind started way back in August. The world, as I knew it, lurched to a halt, and finally, thanks to all of your help and God's grace, it has slowly, but surely, started turning once again.

I've picked my guitar back up after a necessary, but painful hiatus from all things music, and it feels SO good. I can only imagine what the songs I write in the coming months/years are going to sound like and how they'll reflect this whole process, but I look forward to it as much as I'm sure some of you do. For anyone who wants to come out and hear some of the older original tunes and a couple cool covers the band has been working on, we'll be playing a set at Memorial Park a week from Saturday at a fundraiser for Children's Hospital, and we'd love to see you guys there!

Having to face my mortality at such a young age is something I realize many of us don't have to do, but I've seen it as a blessing in disguise. I am incredibly grateful for the growth opportunity I was given, however painful this whole ordeal may have looked from the outside. It definitely put things in perspective. Thank you all again for your continued support. It has meant the world to my family and me. Aloha. :)

Peace, Love, and Edward Sharpe :)

THE WORLD EXHALED!

Life officially became a celebration for us on June 1, about 10 months after Ryder's good news/bad news phone call. We started by visiting the scene of the crime—the cancer center—for a celebration event for survivors. Ryder wanted the whole family to join him, and fortunately, the hospital promised breakfast at 8:00 a.m.

Ryder managed to make it to his world music class orientation, though a bit late. And we headed off to see Reed's matinee performance of THE MUSIC MAN.

Reed lit up the stage and positively glowed after the show. We gave him flowers, which he promptly handed back to me. It had become a tradition to present the boys with a bouquet after their performances, just to have them give it back to take home and put in water. We laughed about that.

Following Reed's play, we dashed to Memorial Park for Ryder's celebratory gig in support of Children's Hospital. Preparing for this brought the smile back to his face and a twinkle to his eye. I wished his nurses could all be there to see the comeback he made, but I knew our community would fill the park.

After Ryder's performance, we hurried back to the high school to catch Reed's evening performance. Somewhere in the midst of it all, Woody packed up to head to Princeton for a month to perform the lead role in SHE LOVES ME.

It was back to the races!

ALLIE

Ryder's Close Friend from Musicians Institute

I went to Pasadena to meet Ryder for dinner and found him playing guitar and singing. As we walked to dinner, we passed a musician performing on the street. We stopped and listened. When he finished his song, Ryder pulled out the money he'd made that night. He gave it to the guy and said, *"Hey man, you need this more than I do."*

I was really touched and said, "Wow Ryder, that was really generous of you." He then flashed that Ryder smile and said, *"Well you can pay it forward and buy me dinner."* And of course, I did.

The Best Gift

Children following their dreams and loving life is what it's all about.

Ryder was happy, planning gigs, tours, and his big trip to Bali for the month of July.

Woody had just left for the East Coast in a flurry of light and enthusiasm with a stop in NYC for what he later called "the best day of my life."

Reed wrapped up THE MUSIC MAN and was on a cloud, racing into finals week with renewed confidence. Awards nights, final concerts, and endless parties were on tap.

Life was good, and I was basking in it.

Our final meeting with the doctor brought continued good news. The markers were all where they should be or better. The past year seemed like an ever more distant nightmare. Ryder's next assessment would come just a week after he returned from Bali. You'd think by now I would have been really good at living in the moment.

Each day brought more openness, more ease, more rehearsals, and more smiles. When the doctor asked how Ryder felt, he replied, *"Grateful. Every day."*

He was looking forward to it all. He had three gigs scheduled before he left in a month. He began commanding the stage, celebrating this life, and serving up joy like slices of cake.

His spiritual life was no longer about seeking it but about living it. He was transforming right before our eyes, emitting a light that was undeniable. He even insisted, before he left for Bali, that Chris and I read Proof of Heaven, which had completely captivated him and fed his belief in God and the connectivity of all things—in life and in death.

RYDER

The good news is that I'm starting to get my hair back after all the chemo and what not. I intend to grow it out, Tarzan length or whatever…ha ha.

Now that that's over and I've been given a new shot at life, I just want to share music—good music—with as many people as I can.

I just want to create a sense of love in the music. It's not about the performer or what you look like up there on the stage. As long as other people are gaining from it and taking a positive vibe from it and they like it, then we're doing our job.

Where I'm at musically is I want to create a sound, with lots of people doing lots of different things. If it's growing and sounds awesome, I just want to build on that and bring as many great aspects into the music as possible that people can jam with.

OLIVER

Ryder's Friend and Collaborator

I don't consider myself a performer. I am way more comfortable in a studio as a composer and producer, but Ryder somehow convinced me to accompany him on stage for a concert. He had a way of making you feel at ease with whatever you were doing, no matter how afraid you were.

As we were tuning up, the owner of a local café kindly offered us a double espresso. It was my first one, but we downed them and then took the stage.

As the audience applauded our first song, Ryder whispered, *"Ollie, you're rushing like heck. I can't sing that fast."* He was serious, but he said it in a way that was filled with humor, love, and grace.

I performed with him many times after that, and I never drank espresso before a show again.

Goodbye and ***

On the way to LAX, Ryder bade us goodbye. *"I love you guys, but I really need to get away (from you)."* He didn't say that, but it hung in the air.

Ryder assured me he'd signed up for free international texting and calling. But surprise! He didn't show up in my contact list. Sigh. Well, I told him to check in with his heart because I would always hear that. Ryder and I had always been psychically connected, finishing each other's thoughts, calling when one of us was thinking about the other.

A timely trip with Reed to see Woody's performances had mercifully left no time to feel the void Ryder left.

Birthday Boy

Ryder's first day in Bali was also his 23rd birthday. As much as I'd have loved to celebrate with him as I had every year of his life, it was fitting that this time he would be on his own, halfway around the world in his personal paradise.

Reed and I went to Princeton to see Woody's play, after which we strolled around the magical campus where princess castles were everywhere we looked. Meanwhile, Chris soldiered on at Disney. I'm sure he was relieved to have us all dispatched so he could work as late as he needed, guiltlessly. I would have felt sorry for him, except that he loved his job so much it could barely be called "work."

We were all connected at the heart, though, and celebrated with Ryder in our spirits.

DARREN

Professor on Ryder's Trip to Bali

I didn't get to meet Ryder until our program orientation for Bali. In walks this guy—late, I might add. I'm silently thinking, "Who is this guy? Man, is he going to be trouble." We started with a round of introductions, and I realized this guy was Ryder—the guy from the emails who'd been going through chemo. So OK, out with my preconceived ideas.

It didn't take long to observe that Ryder was calm, polite, excited to be going to Bali, and a genuinely nice guy. He didn't immediately share the details of his recent battles, but in time the other students would witness how much Ryder was healing and growing.

Everyone and everything made it safely to our villa, with the exception of Ryder's beloved guitar. I knew this meant a lot to him, but after three days of checking with the airline, he came to terms with the loss. He bought a small guitar from a local shop, didn't complain, and didn't let this ruin his experience. That impressed me a lot.

Ryder was at the center of the student group activities. People always wanted to be around him, listening to his stories, his music, and also being listened to.

After a month in Bali, his hair grew in, his skin glowed, and Ryder looked very different from the kid who came to the orientation. Ryder was definitely in a groove, enjoying the "feel" of being in Bali and the rejuvenation in his body.

The girls in the program were very interested in Ryder. Romances developed. Romances ended. Then started up again. It was too much to keep track of, but everyone seemed happy and there was no major drama.

By the end of the program, Ryder was calm, confident, energetic, fun-loving and caring, goofy at times, yet deeply philosophical at others. He enjoyed volunteering at the local schools and having the school children guide us through their village ceremony.

I will forever be impressed by this kid, and I know he's had an impact on all those who knew him.

Two Weeks to Go

Bali was a separation from all things familiar, including friends, family, and habits. It was like sorting through shards of tumbled glass, polished stones, or seashells strewn on a blanket. Some of them he'd unceremoniously toss over a shoulder. Others he would mindfully select as part of a new foundation. I imagined the beaches of Bali as this sorting ground for Ryder.

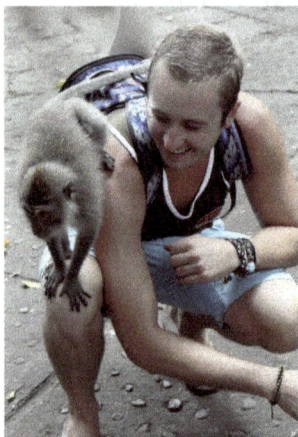

He contacted us only once, and truth be told, I was relieved. This separation was so critical. Otherwise, it would have been like opening the oven door too soon on a soufflé. There would be plenty of time to reconnect and share. I just hoped we'd be able to give him enough room and a clean slate to pin up the parts of himself he chose to bring home.

I needed a break, too. It was a relief not to be tiptoeing around his continuing recovery or wondering about his location. He was under someone else's supervision, and I could finally let go.

I went back to the gym, had lunch with friends, worked on new jewelry designs. And I tended to Reed's and Woody's needs.

Woody had a play in a neighboring community that summer, and we attended every performance. Reed had multiple water polo games every week, some an hour or more away from home. Life was full, and Chris was still working at break-neck speed, trying his best to still be a dad.

Thanks to Facebook, we did briefly connect with Ryder, halfway around the world!

"Miss you guys...Need more money...Want to be Santa when I get home...so much cool stuff... and my phone is drying out in a bowl of rice...may have lost all pictures."

Ahh, all was well. We wouldn't hear much more from him, but knowing he was safe and happy was enough.

ZENA

A Dear High School Friend

We once spent an entire two weeks as couch potatoes, listening to every Beatles song in chronological order. We loved the Beatles as much as we loved each other. They were at the top of a very long list of musicians who had bonded us together. In many ways, I felt like he was my own brother—you know, the one you always wished you'd had.

Ryder shared memories from his time in Bali with me. At the gates of Golden Gate Park there's a welcome sign that was lined with golden poppies. *"In Bali,"* he said, *"They wear flowers in their hair to honor life on earth. I've been doing it ever since."*

Ryder leaned over and picked two flowers, placing one behind his ear and one behind mine. I laughed and asked how many girls he had wooed with this move. He didn't answer, but his laugh told me everything.

After hours of dancing and moving around the festival, we headed home. Ready for bed, I changed into my pajamas and let my hair down. As I brushed through it, I noticed that the little golden poppy had managed to stay there all day. I texted him the good news, and he wrote back that this kept us connected to each other and to the universe. So there we are, Ryder, connected still.

RYDER

You have the power inside of you and in "God" (however you choose to see Him/Her/It). Giving your life up to a power greater than yourself and letting go of the control we try to have in our own lives is the only way to let life truly begin.

There is so much truth in the saying, "Go with the flow;" we have to be willing to stop trying to MAKE things in our life happen and just LET whatever is supposed to happen take place. It takes a serious trust in the Higher Power to let go of it all, but once you do and realize that the things that happen to us are all supposed to and are meant to teach us the things we need to learn, the sooner your life will improve; THAT I can promise you.

Ryder

Welcome Home!

Ryder looked and felt great, except for a little jet lag that had him sleeping for a couple of days. The flower behind his ear and his excitement about Bali's customs notwithstanding, we had to stop at In-N-Out for a burger on the way home from the airport.

As he unloaded a new suitcase full of goodies for everyone, he told us he wanted to move to Bali and make a living teaching English. He had played at every venue possible when he visited, and now he had a following in Bali, as well as job opportunities. If this was what he needed and it would make him happy, I wouldn't object.

Stateside, more tests loomed after the weekend if we could get our insurance company to cooperate. It only approved checkups every six months, which would have launched me into orbit if I weren't confident the doctor would sort it out. Really. Insurance got to decide what was necessary? Sheesh.

I was going back to my "chill" place until the dragon needed to stir. For the moment, it was good to have the whole family together under one roof again.

The Road to Wellness

I was holding my breath, and I'm sure Ryder was, too. What would the tests show? Was he in for more treatment? The trepidation was palpable on the way to the hospital. We chatted a little, but mostly we were lost in our own thoughts.

He got all the necessary blood tests and CT scans, but we had to wait another two weeks for the results.

Ryder wasn't home long enough to share a whole lot with me, but I knew he had a game plan for the next year. He caught a few winks of sleep at odd hours between romps, and he planned to *"get to it"* soon. He ramped up the guitar lessons he loved to give and spent a lot of time pet and house sitting and writing. School would pick up again in January, so he wanted to get one CD done by Christmas and another by next summer. With that, he hoped to save enough money to go back to Bali to teach English and music. This all depended on satisfactory check-ups, of course.

He told me he wanted to do something with children battling the beast. That would probably be the most satisfying of all, and I think he knew that.

I tried to read him on his way in and out the door. Returning to LA was deflating after a month in paradise, and the adjustment seemed grueling for him. I finally learned to let him start the day in his own time. No bright "good mornings" from me.

It was their world. I just lived in it.

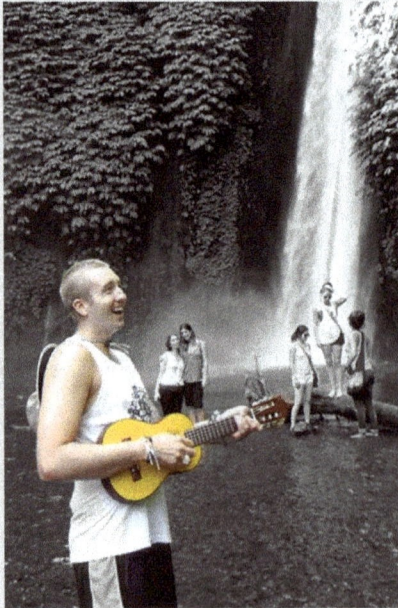

HAYLEY

Friend from Bali Trip

The last day Ryder was in Bali, I sat with him while he cried tears of happiness. He never knew he could be so happy or that he would have been able to be a part of the Bali trip. He was so moved by the experience and so grateful for it. I've never seen anyone look as happy as he did that morning.

All Clear

Ryder's doctor appointment was everything we could have hoped for, and he wouldn't have to go back for another checkup for three months! And so began the waterfall. I could feel myself letting my guard down with tears at every turn. Tears of relief. Tears of gratitude. Tears of joy.

Ryder showed some humility and gratitude, too. Though I could see he didn't really want to dwell on what he had just been through, his visits to the hospital and my profound relief brought it home for him. I was sure that in quiet moments on the hilltops overlooking our community, he thought about it. He could not ignore it. It had shaped him into the man he had become.

He wanted to spend more time with his brothers, realizing how precious this time was. And he focused on the road ahead, while hanging on to the peace he found in Bali. His gigs had a new energy and a lightness that can only come from knowing the dark. It was beautiful to see, even if I was the only one who did.

WOODY

I left to go back to college in Michigan a day or two before Ryder's diagnosis. When I found out he had cancer, I didn't know what that meant. I just knew there was the possibility he could die. I couldn't stop imagining my life without Ryder, and at the same time, I needed to put everything I could into auditioning for shows. I picked a song for my auditions that was about how loving someone is not a choice; it is not in our control—it is why we live. The song ends with:

I will live
And I would die
For you

I broke down and cried during the middle of one of my auditions.

THE ROAD AHEAD

Recovery was more than strong muscles, a tan, and a full head of hair. To look at him, you'd never know what he'd been through or that he was still recovering. It would almost have been easy to put this all behind and try to forget it ever happened. But that would have been to deny the profound changes he and our whole family endured.

A year had been lost, yet not without impact. His world of friends had continued to spin, launching into professional lives or continuing education. It was tempting to flee back to Bali where he had a fledgling fan base and hospitals were a mirage of the past, replaced by soothing waves and swaying palms.

Except for the checkups. He'd have to fly home for those, scheduled every three months, then six months, then? But that was down the road, and relocation to Bali was still just a dream.

The future held many unknowns. But the present had its own problems. His car went belly-up. Like leg-irons, no wheels meant no movement in any direction. That topped the list of all the things to do. School started soon. He needed a job.

So How Was Your Day, Ryder?

As Ryder skipped in from classes in Hollywood, I nonchalantly asked how his day had been.

"Good. Busy. Class. Homework. Reading between classes (sigh). BUSY!" Then as an afterthought, he added, *"Better than sitting around in a bed waiting for the chemo."*

I always asked. I'm sure he sensed there was more to my question than a simple, "How ya doing?" There was. Though cancer was beginning to feel like a bad dream, it was a reality that could land like a bird bomb. Boom. Very Real.

November 11 was our next reality check. With that looming, I had dreams that the cancer was back. I never told Ryder about those dreams. It was far easier for me to bear that alone than watch him endure the thought of his life crashing down around him again.

Had I Noticed Changes?

Yes. There was a carefree easiness and fearless abandon when he played. Finding the light and flowing with it, declaring his dreams and walking towards them without trepidation, giving credit where it was due. He radiated with the great "Not Me."

One experience with him in particular stood out to me.

I joined Ryder and a few of his friends for an ESMZ concert. They continued to be his favorite band, uplifting him spiritually and filling him with just pure love. He ran into several of the band members before the concert, which put him on cloud nine. During the song "Home," the band asked the audience if anyone had a story to tell. Ryder managed to get the mic and shared this story:

> *"You guys saved my life. I've just been through chemother-*
> *apy* (roar from the crowd). *It was hard, but your music,*
> *your vibe, got me through it. I love you all. And I just*
> *want to say thank you. Just, thank you."*

You'd think that would have been the end of a marvelous story, but no. He was invited to join the band backstage and spent an hour and a half connecting with them. Ryder came prepared for this. He told one member he'd written a verse for a specific song where they had a tradition of passing the mic around and band members would improvise a short verse. She said they were going to bring him up on stage and have him sing it the following night. Then she gave him a ticket for that performance.

Ryder connected with them again, and I didn't see him until the next day. His Facebook said they were jamming between shows, so I was holding my breath for the next amazing chapter.

Until then, I was just shaking my head in awe. Without hesitation, he asked for what he wanted and poof! And I thought, "That is how you do it, my boy. You just find the light and go with it because life can be short."

RYDER

Letter to Jade, ESMZ Frontwoman

Namaste!

Hey Jade,

I just wanted to thank you again for being so welcoming and accessible this weekend and for helping me realize the long-time dream I've had of meeting and talking with you and everybody; it was a life-changing weekend for me. Thank you SO MUCH for the music you've made and continue to make. As I've already told you, it truly saved my life emotionally and spiritually, and the chemo took care of the physical.

Keep doing what you're doing; you are amazing at it! You're an inspiration and helped me to find a better way of really living life and living it in love.

I CANNOT WAIT to hear what you've got in store for a solo album, and I'll be spreading it around like wildfire. Really hope we can keep in touch, and I'm sure I'll see you again in the future!

Nothing but peace and love,

Ryder Buck :)

ANDREW

Bandmate

It had been an entire summer since I'd heard from Ryder.

"Hey man it's Ryder. It's super last minute, I know. We're gonna leave in like 20 minutes, but I may have an extra ticket for ESMZ tonight. So I know you'd love to go. Probably got stuff going on, but I just found out. So let me know. All right. Later."

I pulled into the Big Top parking lot, nothing short of jubilant. I heard my name and turned to see Ryder's familiar beaming face. This time there was hair atop his head, which made me smile even more.

Ryder invited me to head to the beer tent with him where we walked around as he unabashedly talked to random attendees. He kept saying how perfect the atmosphere was and how you could feel the love.

"Dude, that was Alex (a.k.a. Edward Sharpe)," I said, stunned, as I watched him walk through the tent.

"What? I'm goin'," Ryder said.

Ryder was on a mission. He was taking the first steps to fulfilling a destiny. He began with declining a handshake for a full hug to which Alex gave no protest.

"Your music means so much to me," Ryder began. He told him the story he gave later that evening during the song, "Home." Alex was moved and departed with thanks and sincere blessings. That encounter and the show itself would have fulfilled the experience for either of us. But little did we know, there was much more to come.

JACK

Grade School Friend

It was only after the show that I learned how important that night was to Ryder. I didn't know the extent of the band's role in fighting back the cancer. I only began to understand when his mom broke down as we watched him share his story to the thousands in attendance.

As the crowd emptied out of the tent, we made our way to meet Ryder by the stage. Thirty seconds later, we were ushered backstage, and Ryder dashed off to get face time with everyone.

For the next hour, he checked in every 10 or 15 minutes, face lit up, working hard not to explode with excitement. At one point, he turned around to find one of the band members walking by. *"Jade!"* He exclaimed, *"I want to jam with you guys!"* Straight to the point. That was his style.

Without any hesitation, she said, "What are you doing tomorrow night?"

That moment stood for what Ryder was all about. His gift was discovering new possibilities. He made you see them and then boldly took steps to make them happen.

Later we ran into another band member, who said his name, "Ryder Buck...Ryder Buck!" three or four times as if reinventing the phrase each time he spoke it. Then he said, "I can't wait to see you fly, Ryder Buck!"

The universe works in mysterious ways.

LESSONS

We honestly did not know how Ryder changed others' lives just by being himself and staying true to his beliefs. As parents, we know that our children teach us more than just about anything else in life, but we never really know the lessons they teach others.

ALEXIS

Ryder's Girlfriend in 2012

Ryder was inspired, creative, and talented, while I had generally become more pragmatic and serious. His romantic and upbeat personality was incredible to be around—in his presence I felt lighter, freer, and happier. Ryder helped me rediscover many important things in life: Being one with nature, expressing love openly, and of course, enjoying good music. One perfect example of this was the evening before I was returning to college; Ryder surprised me with a mini outdoor concert of our favorite songs. It is still easy to picture him standing barefoot in the grass, a big smile on his face, as he strummed his guitar and sang to me.

Ryder's mark on the world is reflected by how many people's lives he touched so deeply. He has left us all with meaningful lessons; he has taught us to appreciate the value of life and to be more generous, loving people. I will never forget the feeling of serenity that I only felt in Ryder's presence. What an amazing gift he was to all who were lucky enough to share time with him.

DYLAN

Ryder's Lifetime Friend

Ryder and I met as babies in Mommy-and-Me gym class and became lifelong friends. We had an unspoken trust and understanding. Ryder was absolutely like a brother to me, except we never fought.

My memories wash in and swirl like waves: the release of Jurassic Park, triggering our fixation with dinosaur taxonomy. Playing the marimba and screeching on the violin, building gingerbread houses and watching for Santa Claus. Our lives were rich and made richer by our companionship.

As we grew older, Ryder's dedication to the guitar was inspiring. He showed me his calluses, and I was impressed by the sudden self-discipline from my usually laid-back, carefree friend.

REED

When my brother passed, it became difficult for me to find joy in just about anything. Life was slow and somber. It was pointless to do anything at all, or so I thought. Until I discovered what comedy was able to do for me. I began watching stand-up comedy specials, funny movies, silly television shows, anything that could possibly make me laugh.

Slowly but surely, I began to chuckle at what I was seeing. The more I laughed, the better I started to feel. I was no longer sulking about my situation and asking the world,

"Why me?" Humor opened my eyes to the harsh reality of life and guided me through the grieving process, a process that I don't believe I would have been able to start were it not for comedy.

I have been studying the art of comedy and analyzing what it is exactly that makes people laugh and why. Comedy is the best gift we have at our disposal, and I can't think of a life better spent than giving someone that gift.

NICHOLE

A Note from London, England

I was at the ESMZ concert the night Ryder shared his story. I never got to meet him personally, but I was utterly moved, transfixed, and inspired by his story and the lessons he had for us all. His spirit, the way he carried himself, the way he spoke, and what he showed us will stay with me forever.

MARCHAN

Fellow Student at Musicians Institute

The first time I met Ryder, I noticed he had an amazing light around him. After my concert that night, he told me I had some groovy licks and called me the guitar girl. Most people who hear my music compliment me on my voice, but I consider myself more of a guitar player. I loved that he noticed that about me first.

The last time I saw Ryder, he was busy writing a song. I wanted to say "hi" to him, but I decided not to interrupt his concentration. I figured I'd wait until next time.

When I found out he'd passed, I went home and immediately started playing my guitar. I didn't know how else to deal with what I was feeling.

My song is about not waiting to talk to somebody until it's too late.

SEAN

Bandmate

My early childhood was spent witnessing a lot of life's ugliness. I can recognize now that I came from a place of privilege, but that doesn't mean things were easy. I didn't have any real concept of home, and Ryder unknowingly gave me the closest thing to it.

I joined Ryder Buck and the Breakers a very pissed-off person, feeling alienated by just about everything and everyone. Through the rehearsals, the jams, the gigs, and the community support, I was able to see a different side of myself and gain a new perspective on my life. Being a Breaker helped heal many of my wounds. It's amazing to think that so much personal transformation took place after a very brief conversation with a guy named Ryder who was simply looking for a drummer.

TAYLOR

Family Friend Through Nikki

Ryder, what a crucial piece of my siblings' musical puzzle you became! If it weren't for you, my brother might have given up on guitar entirely. But you helped him evolve into a man-child guitar demigod. I could always see his eagerness to impress you and pure excitement to jam with you.

Then there's Nikki. It was you who brought the talent out of her. I'm not certain she would ever have capitalized on her potential if it weren't for you asking her to play with your band. You not only helped her grow as an artist, but your passion for it inspired her to create her own.

Ryder Buck, thank you for being our music angel.

NIKKI

Founding Member of Ryder's Band

I first met Ryder at a local jazz night. He complimented me on a song I performed and then asked me to sing backup on his demo track. I remember thinking, "Oh my gosh! He's so much older and so cute, and he's a musician, and he wants me on the track!"

It was the first time I ever recorded anything, and I was super nervous. After that he said, *"Hey, I have a gig. You want to come and sing backup with me next weekend?"* I was thrilled!

I was soon performing regularly with his band. He had a rotating cast of characters, but Ryder was always the heart of it.

We had a conversation one night around the end of his chemo. I remember thinking, "This guy is really remarkable. He's gone through so much and has held his head up high and fought through all of it." His attitude was, *"Cut the bullshit and see that everything is a beautiful opportunity."*

Ryder's repertoire as a musician reminds me of his personality. Each song has a different feel—a little bit of reggae, a bit of blues, some rock and roll. He was an incredible songwriter and an incredible human being.

GRANDMA DOT

One afternoon, Ryder came home and spotted me at the piano.

"Hey Grandma, let's jam!" he yelled.

"Hey, Ryder, you young folks jam. Me, I stick to the music. I've always been a note reader. I've got to have my music. I can't jam, in fact, I don't even know what it is to jam," I said.

"You can do it and I'll show you. First get rid of your music! Now play these notes one after the other with both hands. C-E-G-A-C. Good! Now when I say play, you play these notes and put a little jazz into it."

Sounds easy, I thought, but how can I play without my music?

"Try it, Grandma," he said as he strummed a little tune on his guitar.

I plunked out C-E-G-A-C on the piano. We did this over and over, and I finally gained confidence.

When I heard Ryder say, *"OK Grandma, now we're jamming,"* it was an epiphany for me, although some might just call it jamming!

LAURA

Professor on Study Abroad Trip to Bali

We had a soundtrack to our Bali study abroad program in 2013—and that soundtrack was the voice of Ryder Buck.

He didn't set out to entertain. At first, his playing and singing seemed to just be part of who he was, how he interacted with the world, and the way he processed his experiences along the way.

In 17 years of working with college students, Ryder was unique in his positive nature. Being a young person who had lived through pain, fear, and knowing his own mortality, he came to Bali with an easy, nurturing openness. While he never seemed to struggle to find his place or purpose, he made people around him feel included and comfortable just to be themselves.

DAN

Ryder's Friend

Ryder and I met in junior high. We became close friends because we saw a lot that we admired and respected in each other. Our two groups of friends quickly meshed, and soon we were almost always together.

The summer after high school, we both started working as lifeguards at a local pool. In our last summer there, Ryder and I both had feelings for a girl we worked with, and it strained our relationship. We were too proud to open up to each other, and for the next four years our friendship was never quite the same.

That is, until his last night on earth.

That night, as I clocked out of work, I got a call from Ryder. He asked if I wanted to hang out, so I told him I was about to head to a friend's apartment for a beer. He was obviously welcome and showed up right after me.

We had so many stories to share. He told me about his HUGE dive into spirituality, which dovetailed my own. He told me about meeting his musical heroes, Edward Sharpe and the Magnetic Zeros. It turns out I had met a musical hero of my own about two weeks before his big night. We laughed so hard that we struggled to breathe, and I had never felt so close to him before.

But then my friend John showed up. John and Ryder never really got along. When Ryder and I drifted apart, I grew very close to John. I think Ryder may have been jealous that I'd gotten so close to a new friend. To be honest, I was a little worried because I didn't want anything to spoil the night.

My worries were for naught as Ryder and John bonded instantly. I'd never been so happy to be made fun of. They began cracking playful jokes about me and my quirks, laughing to the point of tears. All I could do was sit back and watch these two who had spent so much time holding onto bitterness just let it melt away and find common ground. They went on to talk about music all night.

Eventually John left, and Ryder and I shared a few more stories before he left. It was October 27 at 2:30 a.m. and I was the last person to see him alive.

When I think of Ryder Buck, I always think of him the way he was that night. So full of optimism, he was ready to throw away a three-year-old grudge with John like it was nothing for a chance to really know someone new. So full of love, he was ready to throw away the bitterness of the past four years of our friendship, hold on to all of the happy memories, and make some new ones. Ryder was so willing to let anyone and everyone become someone special to him.

I thank God every day we buried the hatchet and became best friends again that night.

THE LAST DAY

The last day I saw my beloved son, he spent the night recording and had plans to go back to the studio the following Monday. Then he went surfing and had a private yoga session from which the instructor "had a hard time bringing him back" out of a meditative state. He called me afterward, raving enthusiastically, imploring me to buy him a package of sessions.

He came to Reed's water polo game in Orange County that day. A friend remarked right away he was "glowing." It was good to share the game with him. I knew it boosted Reed, too. Afterwards, as I said goodbye, I looked him in the eye and said, "I love you."

"I love you, too, Mom."

That was it. The last time I laid eyes on him. I'm grateful it was such a poignant moment.

I almost asked him to leave the car and ride back with me, but I didn't. As much as I try now to avoid "what if" moments, that was a big one.

California highway patrol came to our house around 8:30 a.m. My first thought was that Ryder was in jail. But no, he was in the emergency room at a nearby hospital. He'd been in some kind of accident.

My heart began racing and I screamed for Reed, the only other person at home that morning. We were given no further details, and Reed and I were left to fill in the blanks with our deepest fears.

The officer drove us to the hospital where we waited two hours before seeing the surgeon.

I checked my phone during the trip to the hospital. Ryder had tried calling me twice, once at 4:17 a.m. and again at 4:18 a.m. My ringer was off. My ringer was never off, especially when my children weren't home. But I had missed the most important call of my life.

And then there we were, listening to a surgeon painfully recount the many ways my son was broken. In my mind, I was healing them all. We could beat this. We beat cancer. He would heal. Play the guitar again. Laugh. Sing. It would just take time.

But we did not have time. Time was gone. I would never see my son again.

We later learned Ryder was dead on arrival, but through the heroics that ensued, doctors brought his heartbeat back three times. They gave him enough blood for three men. But it didn't save him.

It wasn't cancer that took him. With no warning, he was gone. GONE.

Ryder's car broke down on the freeway on his way home at about 4:00 a.m. He started walking home through a dense fog. It must have been blinding as you still couldn't see three feet ahead by 8:00 a.m. even with the sun fully up. Perhaps, that could explain why he was on the freeway, not beside it. We will never know.

Two speeding cars hit him around 5:25 a.m. Police estimate they were going 75 mph—much too fast.

I had to call Chris in New York City and Woody in London to break the news. Son, brother, GONE. I told Chris that Ryder was "gone." He asked, "Gone where?" My mistake. "Dead" was just too hard to utter.

I don't even remember the call to Woody. He screamed, I think.

REED'S MEMORY

Distant shrieks of pain interrupted the still morning air. I rubbed the sleep from my eyes and hopped out of bed, looking for the source of the sound. As I stumbled down the hallway, I came to the top of the staircase. When I looked down, I saw a police officer standing in front of my mother. She was wailing. The officer told me my brother was in a car accident early this morning and was being treated in the ICU.

Black dots crept into the corners of my eyes as the staircase began to disappear. I couldn't breathe. I felt as if someone punched me square in the chest. My father was in New York for work and my other brother was studying in London; they had no idea what had happened. My mom and I hopped into the squad car and the officer sped off to the hospital.

The waiting room was full of vacant seats. It smelled overwhelmingly of disinfectant. All I could focus on was my mom pacing at the center of the room, wondering what was going on. Left, right, left, right.

The room stood still like a winter morning. Sharp threads of wind found their way through the air vents and began to pierce the grim room. Noise ceased to exist, as if we were in the bowels of a mausoleum. All that was audible was the slow ticking of the clock.

In the distance, a set of steps began to echo. Tip-tap, tip-tap, tip-tap. The steps grew louder, finding their way closer to the room.

I slowly turned my head towards the entrance of the waiting room, hoping to see my brother stumble in. Instead, there stood a man in a white lab coat. He cleared his throat, his lips moved, but my ears seemed to refuse his words. I could see him talking, but nothing seemed to register. It was as if a flash bang had gone off right next to me. A sharp, high-pitched ringing filled my ears.

At 16, I had lost my eldest brother in a fatal car accident. He was a 23-year-old musician who wanted to heal people with music.

Death is a permanent loss. Death doesn't borrow the things he takes. He doesn't return in the morning and restore what he stole. Death is swift and ruthless. The worst part, I thought, was the fear of forgetting who I lost. A voice that once reverberated throughout the house was replaced by soft wisps of wind, a soul fading from existence.

I suppose Bill Watterson had it figured out when Calvin said to Hobbes, "Once it's too late, you appreciate what a miracle life is…nature is ruthless, and our existence is very fragile… it's very confusing. I suppose it will all make sense when we grow up."

WOODY'S MEMORY

I'd just returned to the hostel after a day of touring when I saw a message from my mom. It said, "Call me ASAP." That made me nervous. Why ASAP?

We had trouble getting a good connection, but once we did, she calmly told me what had happened. Ryder was driving home and ended up walking on the freeway after his car broke down. He got hit by two cars and was brought to the hospital where there was nothing more they could do. He was dead.

My immediate reaction was to feel really angry. At Ryder! At Mom. I even started yelling at her until she handed the phone off to Aunt Leslie. This was so unreal, and I couldn't make sense of anything. I just needed details. I needed to know who to blame. Was it Ryder? The drivers? Who were they? Was alcohol involved? Where had Ryder been? Who was there with him?

I started convulsing and crying, and everything was blurry. My friends were there with me, holding me, trying to comfort me as best they could. As lost as I was, I needed details to somehow find my way back from this surreal experience. Being so far from home made it hard to feel the reality of it, let alone the shock of losing my brother.

I made a lot of noise, wailing and yelling, and who knows what else. At one point, my friends decided I needed food, so we set out to find something to eat. On our way to a tapas place, we stopped and bought ice cream. I didn't care if the restaurant got upset that I brought it in. My brother was dead.

I figured since I was flying to Berlin the following day, I'd just fly home from there. Then one of my mom's oldest friends called.

"No, you're flying out tonight!" Another friend had already purchased my ticket. She stayed on the phone with me while I packed and got my ride to the airport.

I was delirious on the flight home. I flew from Barcelona to Istanbul to LA. I journaled a lot during the flights and called friends in between. I was still angry, and I wished I could've hugged Ryder goodbye. It wasn't fair that he did this to us; he couldn't just LEAVE me. I loved him. I didn't know how I'd feel about coming back to my study abroad program after this, and yet that was where I wanted to be. I had so many conflicting feelings, and they made me feel guilty.

On the way home, I just kept thinking about how I wanted to be there for Mom, Dad, and Reed. Once I arrived, I felt like I was living between clouds of grief. It made me cringe to hear the sobs coming from otherwise empty rooms. I still couldn't believe he was gone, and I didn't know how I would be able to handle it. But I was home, and I knew we'd find our way together.

CHRIS' MEMORY

I was in New York City doing publicity interviews for FROZEN. We were taking a quick break when our head of publicity came up to me with her phone. I don't remember if she suggested I sit down, but I found out later that Shelley had recommended I not be alone when I took the call.

Shelley was distraught and told me Ryder was gone. I first thought that he'd been out late and hadn't come home when she expected him—something very common for him. She had to say it several times, finally explaining that he'd been in a car accident and was gone, dead.

I was numb. This couldn't be. Had to be a mistake. But no tears.

Trying to make me feel better, Shelley told me I could stay and finish the interviews if I wanted. Stay?! I knew it was well-intentioned, but I realized she was as off-kilter as I was. In an instant, nothing made sense anymore and all rational thought was gone.

They got me the next flight back to LA. My producer and codirector stayed with me while I packed. Everyone was very concerned about me being alone. Would I collapse and be an emotional wreck? I was too numb for that. And still no tears.

They also offered to fly back with me, but I declined. I just didn't feel like any small talk, even with the people I love. I dreaded the car trip to the airport and the flight itself knowing I'd get the inevitable question, "How are you today?"

Do you lie: "I'm fine. How are you?"

Or tell the truth: "My son died today. I'm a f*cking mess. How are you?"

Luckily, the universe, or Ryder, was looking out for me. Everyone kept to themselves and no meaningless conversations occurred.

I finally made it home and was greeted by Shelley, Reed, and many loving friends and family. I thought once I was home that the tears would flow. Still nothing. Still numb.

I knew sleep that night was going to be impossible. I listened to Edward Sharpe's music, trying to connect with Ryder and hoping it would soothe me to sleep. I finally passed out but woke up in the morning, praying this was all just a nightmare. No such luck.

With the morning being quiet and not many friends at the house, I stole away to Ryder's room and closed the door. I was compelled to be in his space, to try to feel my son, try to feel anything. The numbness lifted and I was overwhelmed with pain—my pain, Shelley's pain, Ryder's pain.

And the tears finally flowed.

A Blur

The house swarmed with friends. The service preparations were launched, woven together with all the elements that had defined Ryder's life: love, music, and inspiration from above.

I grasped at random comforts. Maybe the cancer was coming back and would have taken him slowly and painfully? Snakebite? That was always a possibility on the mountain trails. Shark attack? Plausible. Was it written into his horoscope? Into mine? An astrologer said it was.

Was there pain? A medium said, according to Ryder, *"I was out of my body before the accident happened, watching it like a movie from the side of the road."* I could only hang on to these things as true. What other choice did I have? Absolute despair. Consuming pain. Torture.

The Light Broke Through

I can't imagine how the celebration of life service for Ryder came together just five days later, but it gave our grief a dose of the miraculous before it had really even sunk in.

We anticipated enough people to possibly need an overflow room at the church, but we were not prepared for the 1,200 people who came and stayed for the entire three-hour service.

The biggest shock, though, was the arrival of several members of Edward Sharpe and the Magnetic Zeros, including their front woman, Jade. Having met Ryder a mere week before his death, we were astounded by their desire not only to attend but to perform for us in his honor.

Woody and Reed each sang, Chris sang a lullaby from Ryder's childhood, and Aunt Leslie closed the service the way Ryder closed all of his gigs—by leading everyone in Bob Marley's "One Love."

It was a day of laughter and tears. I even caught myself smiling, especially when Jade led her band onto the altar. I could feel Ryder beaming, laughing in his carefree way, head thrown back.

The Edward Sharpe band was gracious enough to play along with Ryder's band before performing Ryder's favorite song of theirs, "All Wash Out."

I'm grateful for the video of the service because there was no way I could take in and recall all the magical moments that blessed us that day. I was hanging on but only by a thread.

ANDREW

Bandmate

It was unbelievable. Only days earlier, Ryder had told us, *"I'm going to get you playing with them (ESMZ) if it's the last thing I do."* And suddenly we were. And it was.

THE SHOCK WEARS OFF

We are blessed by the mechanism of shock. It dulls the pain and cushions us as we try to adapt to the unacceptable. And then it slowly, gradually wears off.

Chris' movie, FROZEN, launched on Thanksgiving Day just weeks after Ryder's service. That excitement offset our grief, but it was surreal. The highs were so high, and the lows were unbearably low.

Some of our dear friends invited us to share Thanksgiving dinner with them at their house. Alison and Steve were like family to us with three boys about the ages of our own. Alison had been instrumental in pulling together Ryder's service, and she hoped that doing something different than our normal holiday gathering might help.

It did until I stepped out onto their back patio. That had been the scene, just one month prior, of Ryder's last performance. It had been a magical night but reliving the memory of it was too much. I lost it. We stayed through dinner and left immediately after.

That party was the only performance I hadn't recorded. I was full of regrets about that but also grateful that a voice inside me that night insisted I take still photos. They were some of the best photographs I ever took of him with the band. Thank God.

A month after Ryder passed, I remember asking myself, "What is a month? A week? A year?" And the answer was, "Just another undulation in the one long day of my life." Measured in heartbeats. Persistent. Involuntary.

I could not mark time because it all began there—that day—and raised the questions, "Why?" and "What if?" And those questions were a fast pass to hell. There was no future, either. Thoughts of the future brought up the question, "What might have been?" And the mourning soared.

I stopped making plans. I just had the moment. And I was still standing, one breath at a time.

CHRIS

On the career side, things couldn't have been better. FROZEN was getting an amazing response.

On the personal side, things couldn't have been worse. I was a schizophrenic mess.

At Ryder's memorial service, the church was overflowing, mostly with his friends. Friends I'd never met.

Unbeknownst to us, our son had a way of touching people that deeply affected them—even if it was just a one-time meeting. They made a point to tell us their individual stories, and it was clear that he was making the world a better place by giving each one of them hope. And they thanked us.

I was deeply affected by all of this and began to question what I was doing with my life. I was spending most of my waking hours making cartoons.

And then FROZEN came out and became a worldwide phenomenon.

We got letters and emails from people telling us how the film had affected them.

- Autistic kids were connecting to Olaf, some talking for the first time.

- Young adults, feeling isolated because they were different, were now empowered and hopeful because of Elsa's journey.

- More than one talked about being walked back from the brink of suicide.

It became clear to me that I was doing what my son was doing during his life—and what he would have wanted me to keep doing.

But Really God, WHY?

One day soon after Ryder passed, while still in the throes of denial and constant tears, I found myself on the couch, literally shaking my fist at heaven, screaming and sobbing. "WHY ME, GOD? We are a good family! We are kind and generous. We live a good life. Why would you do this to us?"

The answer came: "It just IS. This is your life, now."

"But WHY? You're supposed to be good. There is no goodness here."

God and I had a falling out. We would never see eye to eye on this.

Our family didn't go to church regularly, but I stopped going altogether. Though I still believed in God, there was no reconciling this new reality.

I found myself facing a choice. Give up on life altogether (I implored God to take me) or stick around for my other two sons. I believed at the time they were my only reason to live.

So it became my quest to find the good in life. This took time, but I dove into it. We tried a grief group through the church. Nope. I found comfort on the therapist's couch. He knew the whole family, so this was a good fit. Everyone went once, but I continued to go regularly. There were tears. There was anger, depression, despondency. I unloaded and dragged myself back into life.

I had endless conversations with God, none of them satisfying.

"What is the meaning of this? Where is my son? Was he just on loan?"

"Yes."

Mine for a moment, but never really mine. Just in my care.

God Lent Me an Angel

If I knew then it would be such a brief loan, what would I have done?

I'd have welcomed him as the miracle he was. Which I did.

I'd have loved him with every fiber of my being and measure of my soul. Which I did.

I'd have cherished his sublime smile and his serene demeanor. I did, and I learned from him.

I'd have woken up every time he plopped down on my bed with his guitar in the wee hours. Which, thankfully, I did.

I'd have taken him to that Rolling Stone's concert. Dang.

Careful What You Wish

One morning, I woke up and finally asked Ryder for a sign.

A reporter from CBS called a short while later and said, "I understand you're searching for your son's championship water polo ring. We'd like to help. Can we come up this morning?"

"Um. Sure?"

"OK, let me grab a camera."

Camera? As in, I had to put myself together?

An hour after CBS left, KTLA called.

"6:00 p.m.? OK. Sure."

At least I'd brushed my hair.

It could be said that the ring was just a material thing. I could hear Ryder telling me to let it go.

During our dumpster diving at the California Department of Transportation, I had ignored eye rolls from Chris and Woody and the chuckling of Ryder from somewhere just out of sight, as they helped me rake through debris. I knew they thought I was crazy. But that didn't stop me. I wouldn't stop until I had turned every stone. Every single one.

I had also sent 100 letters to pawn shops all over the Los Angeles area. I did not lack for imagination or stones. And who knows, maybe the added visibility on the news would make them search harder through their inventories.

This was not just a material thing. It meant so much to Ryder. It symbolized the win, which made it a precious trophy. Too dear to wear, Ryder stowed it safely in his top drawer and wore it only on special occasions. Until the cancer.

Then this souvenir became a touchstone for work ethic, built through years of tough-ass, year-round workouts in cold pools at 6:30 a.m. It was about intensity, teamwork, friends pushing each other hard. It meant endurance and digging still deeper when you thought there was nothing more to give. And it meant strength to Ryder, both physical and mental.

Mostly, it was about coming out on top. That was what Ryder saw in his ring, which he wore every day from the start of his chemo. It said to him, "You can do this. Remember what you have already accomplished. Remember what it took to get here. You are stronger than you know."

So when you request a sign, be ready to receive it. He sent me not one, but two TV stations.

"There ya go, Mom. Was that the last stone?"

Maybe we'd see that ring again. If not, it wouldn't be for lack of trying.

Finding Help

Ryder, with Bear and guitar in tow, would hike up a nearby trail, taking in the scenes of our community, downtown skyscrapers, and on clear days, the ocean in the distance. This is where he played his guitar, wrote, meditated, and wooed the girls by starlight.

When he came home, he brought the smell of sagebrush, a bright smile, and the lightness of a fresh outlook.

As a family, we hiked these same mountain trails when the boys were young. They complained the whole way, but we bribed them with the promise of bagels, which completely undermined the benefits of the exercise.

Chris and I hadn't been up there for years until Ryder passed. After that, we made weekly pilgrimages there, dubbing it "Ryder's Peak." It was a place where we could feel his presence and see what he saw.

Hiking to this lofty outlook helped us find the perspective he had: we are all a small part of a very big whole.

> his spirit so big
> Ryder couldn't contain it
> he became the sky

We designed a concrete bench to install on Ryder's peak. The bench was made to look like it was formed from the wood of a tree, and we had it inscribed with the words, "Home is wherever I'm with you," from his musical idols' song, "Home." This bench would never wear away, no matter how many visitors stopped to rest and take in the splendor of this view. Three earth angels, a banker, a contractor, and a surgeon hauled the cement, the water, and the rebar to the top and dug deep into the granite mountainside to install it. I think of Ryder when I'm up there, but I think of them, too.

One morning before dawn, we hiked up to spread some of his ashes. The clouds hung so low that we walked up through them and looked down over them. It occurred to me that this was Ryder's view now. At the very moment we released his ashes, the sun shot a bright orange glow through the clouds. It was a celestial wink, another magical moment provided by my beautiful son.

Too Many Losses

I would continue to get angry with God (again and again).

It was not OK. It was never going to be OK. I had lived my whole life swathed in joy, a grateful awareness of the magic. I could not imagine a life built on a heavy, thick foundation of sadness. A dark fog that never lifted with only infrequent shafts of light breaking through.

This light teased me into believing that there may be whole days, even weeks, of sunshine. Then the fog settled on my shoulders again like heavy bags of sand.

> sadness abounds here
> a blanket covering all
> I peek from beneath

This was the flip side of my life; where there used to be infrequent darkness, now there was infrequent light.

No matter the philosophy, psychic awareness, or belief systems, I lived here, on earth, in a material existence, and Ryder was not here to hug, to hear, to light up the room with his smile. He was gone, not in all ways, but always in some. The world moved around me, and I preferred to sleep.

Unexpected Peace

Peace, like tears, came unexpectedly. Most reliably, peace could be found in the now. Ryder was always striving for that. He talked about it a lot. He appreciated what was right in front of him.

This peace also left me open to Ryder's messages, his presence. I could always feel him when I was grounded in the moment. But it was like walking a tightrope, a delicate balance, easily lost.

One moment I had to face every day was 5:25 a.m., the time when Ryder had passed. I was always awake, and it was torturous for a long time. But when I finally allowed myself to be present in that moment, it began to feel like the most natural time of the day to connect with his spirit. My heart was more open, and it was easier to sense him.

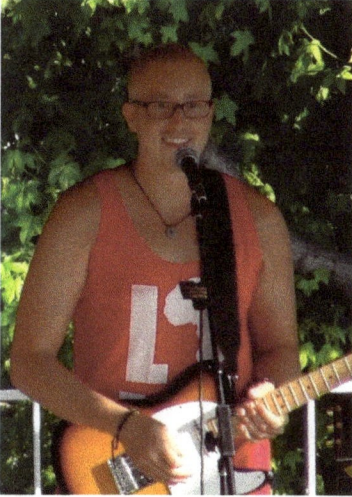

During his chemo, Ryder worked hard to stay in the moment. He didn't want to waste a minute. He even scheduled gigs between rounds and made it a priority to play for the cancer survivors at a local hospital. After Ryder passed, they voted unanimously to give him the hospital's highest award: The Flame of Hope.

Ryder knew what music did for others, and certainly he knew what it did for him. He had a philanthropic heart, which inspired him to use his music to help others. In Ryder's honor, I started visiting Children's Hospital with our therapy dog, Yogi. I only wish I could share his music with the kids, too.

The thing we never forget is that when Ryder passed, he was never happier in his life. He was glowing.

JOACHIM

Band Member

The first time I met Ryder was also my first day at Musicians Institute. We both attended the guitar program and had to get up and improvise a solo. When Ryder got up to play, something hit me. Everyone so far had tried to show off and play as fast as they could and as much as they could. Ryder was not the fastest or the most technical player, but he really said something with his playing.

Ryder came up to me after class and said, "*Hey dude, I really like your playing. We should jam!*" We did, and I ended up playing in his band and he became one of my best friends while I was living in LA.

For Ryder, it was never about playing the fastest riffs or singing the highest notes. It was about getting people to feel something through both his music and his lyrics. That's something I think about to this day whenever I'm on stage or writing a song.

Ryder's band members made regular appearances at our house. His friends came bearing the gift of stories. These were precious moments that kept me anchored in the present. They also kept Ryder close. Forgetting, fading, would be the cruelest cut of all.

I was so grateful for the music he left us and the videos I had religiously taken of their gigs. I was grateful that Ryder's band was enthusiastic about continuing to play together. They sounded better every time I heard them, and I believed there were amazing times ahead for them.

Reed? Ryder?

Ryder's band played at his service with Reed and Woody singing Ryder's vocals.

Immediately after his passing, the band agreed they would keep the full name, Ryder Buck and the Breakers, complete the album Ryder had started, and record more of his original tunes for future CDs.

They didn't want to stop playing together, and, in fact, it was important to each of them to keep Ryder and his music alive. But they needed a lead vocalist. Woody was going back to college. Reed was a trained vocalist with years of experience. He was the obvious choice.

So the band gently and lovingly recruited him to step up and sing his brother's parts. At first, he was hesitant and struggled with the decision every time a performance was looming. Time after time, at the last minute, he'd tell me he wasn't going to do it, which sent me spinning. Venues had been booked, fans notified! Then the band would show up at our house for rehearsal, and he'd somehow rise to the occasion.

I kept scheduling gigs around LA. By now, they had a solid following, filling venues from Hollywood to Malibu.

Months later, during a late-night talk, I had to apologize to Reed. As a mom, my job was to put my children first and protect them. But because it made me so happy to hear Reed sing, hear Ryder's music, and hear Reed singing Ryder's music, I had pressured him silently (and not so silently) to push forward, to "just do it."

I had seen the love, wrapped like angel wings around him, when he was up on stage with Ryder's band. Love from the band members and from the audience, too. I had taken pictures of him beaming, both during and after his performances.

But I knew deep down he wondered if they loved him for himself or as a stand-in for Ryder. It was enough that he saw Ryder in his own reflection in the mirror, that sometimes even he couldn't tell the difference in their voices. Was I asking Reed to bring Ryder back? No. But is that what it felt like to him?

As his mom, I would have thrown myself in front of that train to keep it from hurting him. Yet as a grieving mom, I needed the joy and healing that his performances brought me. Never underestimate the power of grief to offer up the most gut-wrenching challenges and confuse priorities.

Three Amigos

Chris seemed mostly content with solitude, but I needed to have people around me. The empty moments just magnified my loss. Though the daily visits from Ryder's friends helped, they gradually began to trickle off. And then, one at a time, and for different reasons, three of Ryder's band members came to live with us just when I needed them most.

Ryder's other friends were our connection to his childhood and teen years. But Andrew, Trent, and Eddie brought Ryder's music and everything he lived and breathed during his last few years back into the house.

Their joyful, vibrant presence and music soothed our souls. They laughed, teased, and dreamed of the future. And they doted on Reed.

As with most everything, Chris accepted our new house mates with an open heart and a chuckle. We even changed our doorbell ringer to play "Hotel California."

"You can check out any time you like, but you can never leave" (The Eagles).

THE INEXPLICABLE

When we lose someone on the physical plane, things start happening that go beyond our normal reality. And because we're grasping to feel connected to someone we can't see, we're more keenly aware of these things when they happen. They can be lifelines when we're feeling so lost.

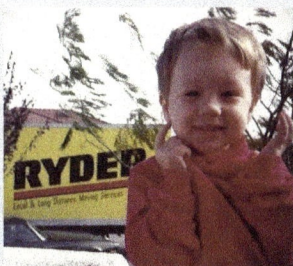

JULIANN

Shelley's Friend

Months after Ryder passed, I went on a cruise with my family. There was no land in sight. I was alone in our room and when I looked out the window, I saw the side of a rusted Ryder truck under our balcony. Right out in the middle of the ocean! I was flabbergasted.

MIKE

An Email from a Stranger

My family and I live in Atlanta, and we recently traveled to Oahu for a Thanksgiving vacation. While snorkeling, we spotted a misshapen object on the ocean floor 12 feet below. We dove down for a closer look and recovered a small brown plastic ukulele. We took our treasure to the beach and emptied the water through the sound hole. As we playfully plucked the strings, we wondered why a ukulele would be at the bottom of the lagoon.

Someone had folded several pages of paper and stuffed them into the body of the ukulele. There were pictures of a boy and a girl with big smiles, enjoying life and one another. Along with the pictures was a 10-page letter that began with the words, "Dear Ryder." We carefully peeled each soggy page apart and continued reading. The letter led us to the assumption that this must be a young lady's breakup and final goodbye letter. It included references to him having cancer, such as, "Why did it happen to you?" and "We will be better together in heaven."

We realized that this was much more than a simple breakup letter. We were conflicted. Our better judgment and conscience was telling us to put it all back as we found it. Yet, we had a deep curiosity to learn more about their story and maybe why this came onto our path.

The letter mentioned his playing guitar and having a band. I, too, have been in a band for many years, and one of my first instruments was a small brown ukulele. A young man traveling with us was also a guitar player who had battled his own cancer.

We needed to know more, but the letter revealed very few clues: a guitar player, a romantic memory of a time at LC golf course, and another at Sugarloaf.

When we searched one of my musician websites, Reverb Nation, we found 500 artists named Ryder. We began comparing the wrinkled paper photographs to the artist pictures on the site. On the third click, we spotted a young man with similar looks holding a guitar with his back against a rock at the beach. A few more clicks and we were delighted to see the pictures matched! Ryder Buck from La Canada Flintridge, CA. There was the LC and, yes, there was a Sugarloaf not too far away.

We enjoyed listening to his music and felt as if we somehow knew him. From there, we visited his Facebook page and discovered even more of his appetite and love for music. We saw pictures of a wonderful, spirited life.

We googled "Ryder Buck Musician." The top of the page returned the words I suppose we feared but quietly expected. In the month prior, after completing chemotherapy and returning to the Musicians Institute, Ryder died but not of cancer.

The identity of the young lady who authored the letter remains unknown, and her questions "why" will also likely remain unanswered. However, we have answered with certainty that a person's spirit and his music can reach across thousands of miles and live forever, without question.

MARY

Ryder's High School Girlfriend

I was in love with Ryder. However, in the middle of my freshman year of college we officially broke up. We still loved each other, but we had to let each other go so we could grow up.

Our breakup was painful, but I immersed myself in my college athletic career. My goal was to be a great volleyball player, and I was convinced that this would bring me true happiness.

I worked hard and was becoming the volleyball player that I had aspired to be. On Saturday, October 26, I played the best game of my career. Little did I know that within hours my world would change forever. I remember the moment well. I was outside a sandwich shop when I checked Facebook on my phone. I saw the words, "RIP Ryder Buck." I was in a state of shock. Moments before, I was so happy about accomplishing a goal that seemed so important. Now I felt the deepest pain I had ever felt. I kept thinking this had to be a mistake. We had just texted each other and he was so happy. How could he be gone so quickly?

We were heading to Hawaii for a volleyball game, and I knew this would be the perfect place to honor Ryder. On my flight over, I wrote my last love letter to him. The more I poured into this letter, the more it made me realize the sweet and tender nature of our relationship. It was the purest form of love I had ever experienced.

Writing also enabled me to realize how unhappy I was with the person I was becoming. I felt like I was living my life robotically without passion and love. It was time for me to create a life filled with the kind of love that Ryder had taught me, so I decided to break up with the guy I was dating. He wasn't treating me well, and he definitely didn't measure up to what I had known.

When we landed, I bought a ukulele. I loaded it with my letter and pictures of us together. At five o'clock the next morning, my mom and grandma joined me to watch the sunrise. I talked to Ryder, told him how much I loved him, and threw the ukulele into the ocean.

I often wonder if Ryder was an angel even when he was alive. Though my heart broke into a million pieces when he died, his spirit gave me the courage to pick up those pieces and become the person he knew I could be.

MESSAGES

A dear friend called me from across the country and said, "I think Ryder really wants me to tell you to *'Leave your light on.'* Does that mean anything to you?" She knew it was the title of a song he had written, but she wondered why she couldn't get it out of her head. I knew exactly why.

Just the day before, I turned off his lava lamp. It had been running since he passed. For some reason, I thought I should be able to do that, but it felt so symbolic it was disturbing. Then when I got her message I thought, "Ok, well, whether that was meant literally or it was just a *'Hey Mom, I'm here,'* it really doesn't matter because he contacted me!" I turned the lava lamp back on.

Ryder's Visit

HE CAME! Oh, my gosh! HE CAME!

Sleeping soundly with Chris purring softly beside me, I had an encounter with my son.

I knew when it was happening that I would only be able to describe this as a "dream," but it felt like more than that. It was like a state of consciousness within a dream. Very real.

I heard his distinctive voice and looked up with a start. Was that RYDER? I saw only his legs as he disappeared into the studio. I flew after him. There he was! The biggest, longest, warmest hugs ensued.

"NOW you like my hugs. Ha ha."

"Silly, I've always loved your hugs."

He had two friends with him, a guy and a girl. They put on a light show for me.

"Get this, Mom."

He put on headphones, and they spun into balls of light with electric blue neon-like threads running through them and sparkles swirling through the air.

"Is that hard to do? Does it take a lot of energy?" I asked.

"Nah, just some practice. Ha ha."

I apologized for the ways I had failed him. He looked a little sad but shrugged it off.

As Ryder was preparing to leave, his guide, a woman in white who hadn't been with us so far, gave him a washer-like coin with a pink sticker on it to give to me. It dropped, rolled away under a car, and we couldn't find it. We tried to find a replacement but couldn't, and I thought, "Oh well, it's just a token. I have the visit."

Was this a symbol for the ring?

SUE

Family Friend

In a dream Ryder told me he was met on the other side by a lot of people who already knew him. One was *"a really spiritual guy"* whose name was John. We figured out later that Chris had an Uncle Bud who was really named John. He was a Jesuit priest at the Biblical Institute in Rome. So Uncle Bud, a.k.a. John, had met Ryder.

Then Came Oscar

Two months into the New Year came the Oscars. The movie was a smash hit, confounding us all with its scope. It was surreal. Blinded by grief, I found it hard to keep up with the celebrations.

When the awards season came, FROZEN swept through them, culminating in the big one, Oscar, himself. We won in two categories that night, and as Chris thanked the powers that be, he also thanked "our guardian angel, my son, Ryder Buck." Just as he said Ryder's name a light flashed across his codirector's dress.

I could instantly see Ryder, laughing in his light-hearted way, blessing our daily endeavors.

Another Gift from Above

Ryder was carrying his laptop the night of the accident, and it was no easier to fix than he was.

One night, muddling around on my computer, I found the tracks from the last recording session of his life.

Because the computer specialists had been unable to retrieve them from his laptop, we thought they had been lost forever. And though there was no explaining how they showed up on my computer, we now had clean, separate tracks for three more songs. This was nothing short of a miracle!

That night, I was able to rest and listen to the rain feeding the wildflower seeds we had scattered up on Ryder's Peak. If they hadn't been washed into the ocean, we would have color soon.

RETRACING HIS STEPS

Occasionally, Ryder sends messages through a friend, who receives them like a fax. She wakes up at night, transcribes them, and then sends them to me the next day. This one came in June of 2014 just before our first trip to Bali:

Dear Mom,

Happy Belated Birthday, ha ha...

I wanted you to know how excited I am that you are going to Bali! The people are the kindest and most loving people any-where, and they are magical.

The trip will be overwhelming for you, but I needed to remind you to please be happy. You might be tempted to be sad when you visit all the places where I stayed, played, and just had great times.

Just allow yourself to experience the range of emotions. Just go with the flow. If you cry, that is OK. Let yourself cry. It is really important to me that you ALLOW YOURSELF TO BE HAPPY, too!

I will be there with you THE WHOLE TIME!

I love all of you, and I am so happy! I am always with you!

Love forever to infinity!

Ryder

Ryder's Appearance in Bali

In the early months after Ryder passed, we were in touch with the professors who chaperoned his class to Bali. It didn't take long for us to decide we wanted to follow in Ryder's footsteps, and these were the people who could make it happen.

Gathering our closest friends, those who had known Ryder since infancy, we planned our two-week trip for the summer of 2014, exactly one year after he was there. The Gabriels from our Disney family, Karla who taught his first Mommy-and-Me gym class, and her son, Dylan, whom I considered one of my own, all banded together in anticipation of the experience of a lifetime.

We knew there would be mystical experiences ahead. As we retraced his journey towards what I now came to think of as enlightenment, we were on heightened alert for his signs and signals.

The first night we arrived, Karla had a dream. She was in a cab, riding through the streets of Ubud. On an alley just off Main Street, the driver pointed out an open-air pool hall. He asked Karla if she wanted to go in. She said, "no." Then back on the main street, she saw a blond boy about nine years old staring at her. "Ryder? Is that you?"

"Yes, it's me."

She told the driver to stop the car. Ryder got in.

"I'm so happy that you are all here. I'm having so much fun with you all here. Are you having fun?"

"Yes, we're having a great time."

Then the driver said, "Who are you talking to?"

And Karla realized he couldn't see Ryder.

Karla told me this story the next morning at breakfast. That night, we went into town for dinner. Stuck in traffic, I saw an old Western-style sign that said, "Pool. Darts." I pointed it out to Karla, and she said, "Yes, but in my dream, it was open-air. No door." As we drove on by, we saw that the entrance was up a little alley off Main Street, and it was open air!

We stopped to take a closer look, and then I saw the pool tables. There he was! A young man with a peach-fuzz halo of hair just like Ryder's hair looked when he left for Bali last year and wearing the glasses I loved so much.

Time stopped. I stared, waiting for him to move. He stayed in that position for several seconds, long enough for Karla to take a picture. Then he turned towards us, and it was someone else.

Coming Home

After returning from Bali, I became contemplative in a whole different way. I had experienced many mystical encounters with Ryder and knew a great deal of healing had taken place.

Gathering photos of my three boys together, I saw a theme emerging: A serene Ryder, somewhat apart in spirit and energy from the two exuberant clowns beside him. Woody and Reed were fully engaged with the camera as if to say, "Look at me!" But Ryder seemed more like a tree, a sublime presence saying, *"I see you."*

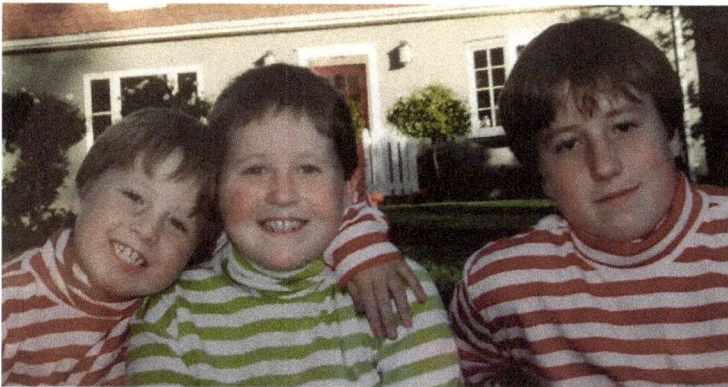

KEEPING HIM ALIVE

In the early days after he passed, I remember how much solace I got from looking at photos, watching videos, and listening to the music Ryder recorded. This was where I went when I didn't know what else to do with myself. It soothed me and it kept him close. This didn't work for Chris and others in my family, though. As we learned through this loss, we are all different in terms of what brings the healing we need.

One thing we all did agree on was the need to establish a Ryder Buck Memorial Scholarship at his high school. Ryder gained so much confidence and encouragement during his time there, and we felt compelled to give back. In addition to encouraging and supporting other young musicians in their early development, we also wanted to ensure that the recipients felt a kinship with what Ryder was about and that they were committed to sharing their gifts with the world.

We had a successful benefit concert to raise money for the scholarship where his band, Ryder Buck and the Breakers, performed. Orbs of light shot across the stage, which showed up in the video I shot that night. There were no disco balls in the place, so guess whose light it was?

Learning to See My Own Light

When Ryder came into the world, I was in my mid-thirties, an impatient, intense, creatively driven person with no limits to my optimism. He slowly softened my edges, making me think more about how my energy was affecting others, but the optimism stayed.

Until he died, that is. I thought I'd never find it again, but I gradually learned to let Ryder's light lead me forward.

It started with a trip to a tattoo parlor. Ryder had returned from Bali with a tattoo on his forearm, which he knew I wouldn't like. He passed it off as *"temporary,"* while I rolled my eyes and he smirked.

The tattoo was the Balinese symbol for Ohm, the sacred sound of the universe.

After he passed, I found myself leading a group into a local tattoo parlor. My attitude had completely changed. Now I saw putting this permanent symbol on my body as something I would proudly display for the rest of my life. This was my first tattoo, and it would be my last.

My mother, sister, sister-in-law, and two band members were lined up behind me. Grandma Dot, at 84, became their oldest customer.

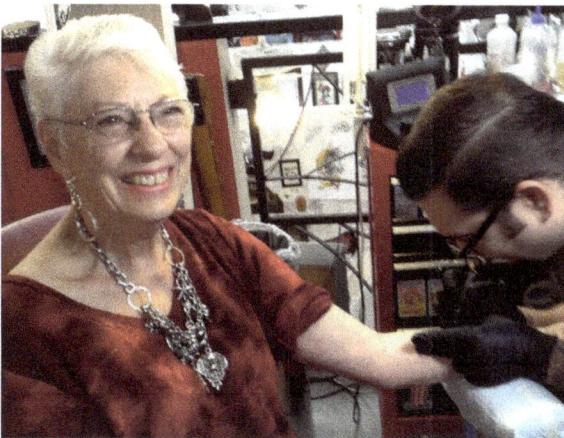

This tribute put us all in greater touch with Ryder and helped us appreciate some of what he had been practicing in his own life: To meditate, see God in the everyday little things, and be in the moment. It also gave us the comfort of sharing our grief with each other, and it felt like a hopeful act.

Whether in dreams, intuitions, or tangible events, Ryder's light was always there. I wasn't very experienced with the mystical side of life, but

I couldn't deny that some of what was happening to me was coming from him. Like the night I had this dream about him:

> Ryder came home with a rescued puppy. Very uncharacteristically, I said he had to go back. Ryder started to weep, which was a sign I had gotten it wrong, again. He protested, *"If I take him back, they'll put him to sleep."* I did a quick reverse and said we'd keep him. Ryder brightened up.

The morning after my dream, I got a text from a friend who had just rescued a stray. He was matted, full of fleas and ticks, and scrawny. They had named him Chance. Thanks to the dream, my heart was open, and I said, "Bring him over!"

We gave the little guy the second chance he needed, and I got one, too. More healing for me and a forever family for Chance. I could feel Ryder smiling.

As time moved forward, I continued to choose Ryder's light over the darkness that grief brought. I thought about his rebellious spirit, his goofy ways, his belief in the power of a loving and open heart, and I began to let go of my pain. I contemplated my life more deeply. I felt realism replace my optimism, and patience moved in where impatience used to live.

My son has changed me. He didn't worry about getting things perfect. He barely worried, period. Though he did contemplate the meaning of things and followed his passions from within his young and messy heart.

If I can leave half the imprint on life that he did, I will be thrilled. If I can help his light continue to touch and encourage others to be who they really are, that will make me happy.

The world needs more of that.

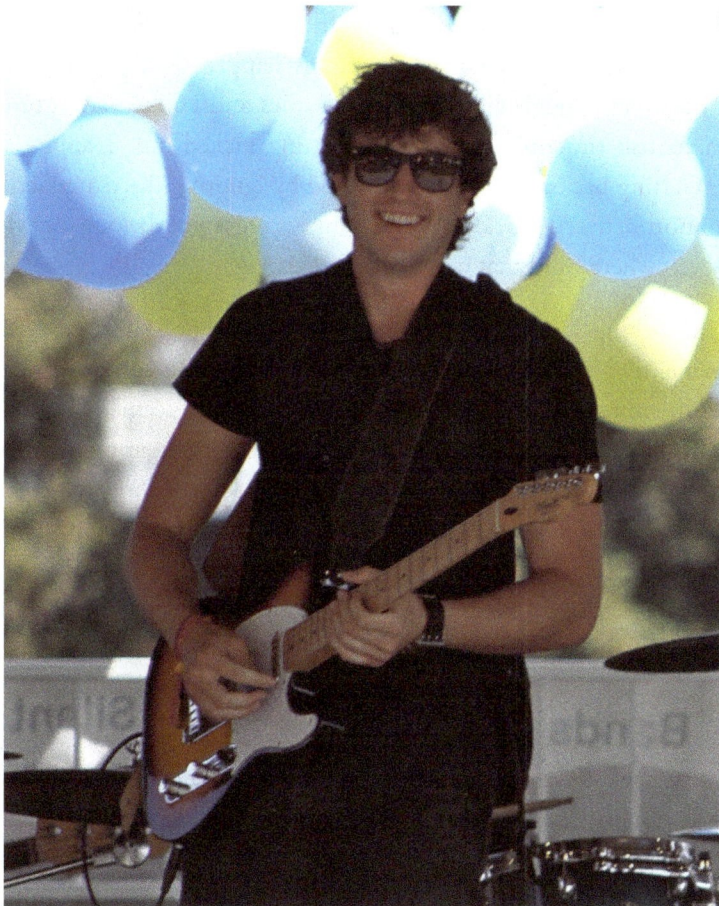

AFTERWORD

I first noticed Ryder backstage at our five-day Big Top show we held under a circus tent. How he and his friends made it backstage I don't know. You never know how these things happen, you just appreciate that they had enough disregard for the rules and enough adventure in them to risk the embarrassment of getting kicked out. I appreciated that. Getting backstage is also predicated by ignoring the manufactured separation between "rock star" and "fan," a sense you belong anywhere and everywhere. And that was Ryder Buck.

The first thing I noticed about him was his smile. His face seemed permanently hijacked by the kind of smile that knows some spectacular secret the rest of us are about to learn. His friends all seemed to have the same smile on their faces, but all seemed to attribute their own smiles to Ryder's. One of his friends came up to me, wide eyed, not to lather me in praise, but to talk up Ryder. It was then that I picked up on Ryder's history and victory over cancer, a magical and mystical feat, as I always view such victories. Of course, I was in some hurry, rushing to rush to get on stage, and I lost them in the madness soon after.

But then I saw Ryder again. And then again.

The first "again" I recall as a blur and would be hesitant to speak on were it not for the fact that I only saw him thrice and so each time counts. It was a part in the song "Home" in which we ask the audience for stories and hand them the microphone. This memory is as fuzzy as the intoxication of music itself, but I recall finding Ryder in the crowd and handing him the mic. He told his story of recovery from cancer. I remember his smile, still, and the Big Top crowd all a'hugged for him.

The next "again" was just outside of the tent the following night. Someone was singing one of our songs, "Jangling," with a guitar. It was Ryder. He was standing alone, guitar in hand, singing full-throated and in earnest—and smiling. That is the moment I think of most for two reasons. It was the last time I saw him, and because I felt his singing was an open invitation, one which I, likely because of my own self-consciousness, did not embrace. "There will always be another time, surely." But then there wasn't another time. That was it. And that sticks with me. That moment. That invitation by someone brave, to be brave with them. To sing. To smile. To live in earnest. That seemed, to me, to be Ryder Buck.

ALEX EBERT, a.k.a. Edward Sharpe of
Edward Sharpe and the Magnetic Zeros

"Leave Your Light On"
by Ryder Buck

https://www.youtube.com/watch?v=9svuc587DOA

Rollin' out
With the tide
And girl you're all that's
On my mind
Leave your light on baby
Yeah, leave your light on baby (echo)
Leave your light on baby
You know my loving's free
If you just leave your light on for me
Eyes green like
Ocean waves
See me through those
Longer days
Leave your light on baby
Yeah, leave your light on baby
Well, you know my loving's free
If you just leave your light on for me
Babe I'm comin' on
Home to you
I know you'd never ever
Be untrue
Leave your light on baby
Yeah, leave your light on baby
You know my loving's free
If you just...
I said my loving's free if you JUST...
Girl, my loving's free if you just...
Leave your light on for me.

Ryder Buck's music is available on Amazon, iTunes, and Spotify.

"Leave Your Light On" Ryder Buck

"Life After Life" Ryder Buck & the Breakers

"Three of Three" Ryder Buck & the Breakers

RyderBuckMusic.com

ACKNOWLEDGEMENTS

We chose to share our story because of what our son taught us about living large, even when the magnitude of our experience made us feel terrifyingly small. We had no idea where things would go when this all began but staying connected kept my family and our amazing circle of friends strong when the journey became inexplicable.

There are people to whom I owe special thanks, those who traveled these roads with us and rounded out our nuclear family with their doting hearts.

Dr. Brown, who found the cancer.

Dr. Quinn, who treated us both with a deft touch.

CaringBridge.org, a free, interactive website where people in the throes of a health crisis can share updates with friends and family. It became my catharsis, my therapy, and the basis for this book.

Coach B for introducing me to CaringBridge.org. From the moment he heard of Ryder's diagnosis, he was there looking out for Reed, and also for me. Ryder was a championship player on his water polo team, and Reed was following suit.

Kathy Curtis, my oldest and most trusted friend, for taking my thoughts and forming them into this book. Her magic and intuition are the sparkle and glue that hold this story together.

Katherine Kavich for her recommendations, encouragement, and enthusiastic support.

Pete Donaldson for his interest and guidance in getting these precious memories into shape for publication and beyond.

Chris, Woody, and Reed Buck, who were always there, born into their roles, as father and brothers.

Grandma Dot, who stood in for me from the crib on.

Aunt Leslie, who redefined "aunt" in all ways.

Karla, Alison, Teryl, Tammy, and the Gabriels, who formed the village in which we raised our brood.

Ms. Rios, who made it cool for a water polo player to sing on stage.

Alex Ebert of Ryder's favorite band, Edward Sharpe and the Magnetic Zeros, and

Jade Castrinos, formerly of the same band, for welcoming Ryder and making one of his life's dreams come true.

The members of Ryder Buck and the Breakers; Nikki Segal, Cameron Wehrle, Jø Henrixon, Sean Moriarity, Andrew Avitia, Eddie Haddad, Trent Carroll, Sean Segal, Oliver Schnee, Woody Buck, and Reed Buck.

They brought his music to life and carried his love to the stage.

The muses, who inspired his love songs.

The children of Bali, who tickled his imagination.

All the loving souls, who contributed their own stories and let us see the Ryder they knew.

Our community of friends and family, who fueled his light and feel it still.

Shelley Buck

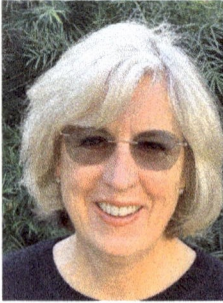

Shelley Buck was born into a creative family in the Midwest and moved to California after college to follow her dream of working for Disney. It was there she met and fell in love with her husband, Chris, who worked in animation. After they married and had their first child, Ryder, she stayed home to be a full-time mom to him and the two brothers who followed.

She is a storyteller and artist, which she expresses through her original jewelry at ShelRae Designs. When Ryder was diagnosed with cancer and the journey went to unimaginable places, she poured her heart into writing their story. Her lessons in parenting through these tribulations, combined with the power of Ryder's larger-than-life spirit, offer profound messages for living in the light.

Kathy Curtis

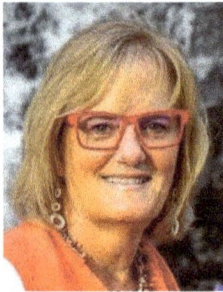

Kathy Curtis moved into Shelley's neighborhood when they were both 12 years old and an instant, lifelong friendship took root. She has worked as a healing artist and writer since 1991. Her programs support the transformation of grief, illness, and emotional barriers through creative expression. She is the author of *Invisible Ink*, a memoir about her own journey through grief. The unique writing process that brought her so much healing has since become a successful program, online and at various venues in the Midwest.

Kathy's intimate connection to the Buck family, combined with her writing and healing background, made her the perfect person to partner with Shelley on the creation of this book.

www.ingramcontent.com/pod-product-compliance
Lightning Source LLC
Chambersburg PA
CBHW060319030426
42336CB00011B/1118

* 9 7 8 1 7 3 4 4 8 4 4 0 3 *